Contemporary Medical Ethics

Contemporary Medical Ethics

JOHN F. DEDEK

SHEED AND WARD, INC.
Subsidiary of Universal Press Syndicate
New York

 For information write Sheed and Ward, Inc. 475 Fifth Avenue, New York, N.Y. 10017.

Library of Congress Catalog Card Number 75-1661
ISBN: 0-8362-0617-7

As a stream cannot rise above its source, so a code cannot change a low-grade man into a high-grade doctor, but it can help a good man to be a better man and a more enlightened doctor. It can quicken and inform a conscience, but not create one.

International code of Medical Ethics, adopted by the General Assembly of the World Medical Association, London, 1949.

CONTENTS

FOREWORD

The last few decades have witnessed extraordinary developments in the fields of science and medicine. The discovery of DNA and the cracking of the genetic code strike at the very origins of life and open the doorway to genetic planning. Organ transplantation is being mastered and the selection of suitable donors and recipients is creating massive problems.

In the field of sociology the demographers' warnings of food and energy shortages due to burgeoning populations have begun to be substantiated. The excesses in human experimentation during World War II have resulted in the Declaration of Helsinki, which states the rights of the individual and has been confirmed by most governments.

These rapid developments have required the Catholic Church to reconsider its teachings and role in all areas where ethics are concerned. Traditionally this burden has fallen on the moral theologians and, ultimately, on the Pope. Vatican II was called in an effort to update the Church and adapt it to the twentieth century. Since then, and in the face of increasing knowledge, absolute statements regarding right and wrong are no longer acceptable in the face of increasing knowledge. This was clearly exemplified by the debate and controversy that followed on the publication of *Humanae Vitae*, a response which has threatened the magisterium of the Pope..

The modern physician, Catholic or non-Catholic, whatever specialty he pursues, has constantly to make decisions involving ethics and morals. In this rapidly changing world with its facilities for instant communication there are few concise and up-to-date sources of knowledge in the field of ethics to which he can refer. Father John F. Dedek has attempted to supply this need in his *Contemporary Medical Ethics*. This has not been an easy task in view of the breadth of the matter and its controversial nature. The difficult problem areas are discussed well with appropriate references. Official Church teaching is presented, along with the most contemporary theological opinion. The two do not always coincide. But it is important that all views be presented in a modern textbook, lest it amount to nothing but a rehash of outdated material. This book will be a valuable addition to all hospital and medical school libraries.

William P. McKeever, M.D.
F.A.C.P.
Associate Professor of Medicine
Northwestern University
University Medical School
Chicago, Ill.

Part One

The Human Body

CHAPTER **1**

SURGERY

A physician who took the Hippocratic oath in its earliest form swore to leave surgery to the surgeons, men especially skilled in the use of the knife. "I will not use the knife," he vowed, "even on sufferers from stone, but I will give place to such as are craftsmen therein."[1]

In modern American hospitals the skill of the practicing surgeon is guaranteed by more than the Hippocratic oath. It is guaranteed by the American Commission on Accreditation of Hospitals, which is made up of representatives of the American Medical Association, the American College of Surgeons, the American College of Physicians, and the American Hospital Association.

To obtain accreditation every hospital must meet high and rigid standards and must accept only ethical and qualified surgeons as members of its staff. After graduating from medical school and serving a general internship of one to two years, a doctor begins his surgical residency, which in most good hospitals extends over a period of five to six years. Only when he has successfully completed this period of training—at about the age of thirty-two—is he allowed to begin private practice. And even then his hospital may not allow him to perform major surgery without the supervision of some older and more experienced member of the staff.

Nonetheless, it is not an adequate statement to say that good surgery is good morality. There are ethical issues which lie beyond the reach of this simple statement. Given that the surgeon is a highly skilled craftsman and given that the operation under consideration almost certainly will be successful, it is not necessarily clear that the operation ought to be performed.

Take, for instance, the case of a spina bifida with a meningomyelocele. This presents as difficult a moral issue as there is. Richard McCormick described the problem in this way: "Prior to the mid-1950's, few babies born with this defect survived for very long. Hence the moral problem was not terribly urgent. Now, however, advances in medical knowledge and technology make it possible through surgery to prevent further contamination of the spinal fluid and lethal infection. If surgery is not performed, the infant will probably contract meningitis due to bacterial invasion of the open sack of spinal fluid and die. However, the surgical prognosis is highly variable. Sometimes it is quite poor. At other times, it is good, but even with a fairly good prognosis, these children can end up severely impaired and in a constantly deteriorating condition which represents a tremendous burden on the child and his family. For instance, in many of these cases nerve function is impaired from the defect downward, so that the child cannot walk without the aid of crutches and braces. Even to walk with crutches requires extensive physical therapy that continues throughout the life of the child. In 90% of these cases hydrocephalus develops. With immediate treatment by surgical insertion of a shunt (a tube which drains the cerebrospinal fluid from the brain into the heart and peritoneum) the child still has a 50-50 chance of being mentally retarded—and the shunt may need revision several times. Without such a shunt the infant will definitely be retarded and could quite possibly die as a result of intracranial pressure. Even if hydrocephalus does not develop, there is no guarantee that the child will not suffer some degree of mental retardation. Furthermore, this condition is not infrequently associated with lifetime loss of bladder and bowel control. The instance is complicated by the fact that the decision must be made within hours of birth if optimum results are to be had; but even at this optimal time it is difficult to predict its ultimate outcome."[2]

Notice that here the question is not about someone who is caught up in the irreversible process of dying but about someone whose dying process can be reversed and whose life can be saved in most instances. Prompt and skillful surgery quite likely will save the child for a crippled, painful, and retarded existence. And so the moral question is whether skillful and effective surgery really represents the most human and Christian choice. In this instance is that which is medically indicated also morally indicated? Is good medicine also good morality here?

If we judge that surgery should not be performed, that it should be omitted in this case with only supportive care provided to the child until it dies, then we are implicitly making a judgment about the quality of life that is worth living. To judge that the diminished quality of the life that the child will have is reason for not saving it may be morally appropriate or not. But it is a distinctively moral question which goes beyond the canons for good surgery.

We will discuss this and similar issues in a moment. But first we need to take a look at some of the principles and language that moralists use in their efforts to illumine ethical decisions in this area.

The Principal of Totality

The ethical principle which finds application in every

surgical operation has been formulated by Bruno Schüller. It states that physical (or premoral) evil becomes moral evil only when it is done without a proportionate reason. An amputation, laparotomy, colectomy, and so forth are in themselves quite clearly physical evils. To perform them for no good reason would be morally evil as well, the sinful violation of a person's bodily integrity. But if an organ is diseased and presents a threat to the whole organism, as, for instance, a gangrenous foot or a cancerous colon, it is reasonable and morally right to excise it. Similarly, if a laparotomy is performed for necessary abdominal exploration or surgery, it is morally good, since there is a proportionate reason justifying the physical mutilation that occurs.

Our common moral sense intuitively makes such practical judgments without any difficulty. It instinctively recognizes that the ancient and elementary medical principle, *primum non nocere* (first of all, do no harm), needs an immediate qualification, i.e., do no harm unless it is necessary to achieve a greater good.

Moralists long ago formulated reflexly a moral principle that is implicitly at work in any practical decision to do surgery. In the thirteenth century Thomas Aquinas put it this way: "Since any member is part of the whole human body, it exists for the sake of the whole. . . . Hence a member of the human body is to be disposed of according as it is beneficial to the whole. Per se a member of the human body is indeed useful for the good of the whole body; per accidens however it can happen that it is harmful, for example when the member is diseased and corruptive of the whole body."[3]

This Thomistic doctrine came to be known as the principle of totality. Simply put, it affirms that since the part exists for the sake of the whole, it may be sacrificed for the good of the whole. The principle gradually was assimilated into Catholic medical ethics, and during the pontificates of Pope

Pius XI and Pope Pius XII it became part of official papal teaching.[4]

The principle of totality does not assert that only diseased organs may be surgically removed. Even healthy organs may be excised for the good of the whole. For instance, healthy testicles or ovaries may be removed in order to prevent the spread of cancer. Or a healthy appendix may be removed as a precautionary measure when the abdomen is already open in the course of another surgical operation.

Also, the principle of totality does not demand that the surgery be truly necessary. It only requires that it be genuinely useful to the patient. A cholecystectomy for a gall bladder ailment, for example, is a reasonable and moral choice even though a man could keep the condition under control by going on an heroic diet. Surgery is morally justified when it offers a person sound hope of genuine benefit and when this same benefit cannot be obtained by simpler means that are reasonably available.

Finally, it is not just the good of the whole body that justifies surgery. It is the total good of the person. Therefore, cosmetic surgery is also justified by the principle of totality. Thus, while plastic surgery done to enlarge small breasts contributes nothing toward the physical health of a woman, it may be very beneficial to her psychological or emotional well-being. Similarly, an infant born with an extra thumb on each hand would have more efficient hands than the rest of us, but the physical advantage would be offset by the probable psychological effects of being anatomically different from the rest of the human race.

The principle of totality affirms that a person's stewardship over his body includes a natural right to dispose of its members in accord with his overall good. It excludes on moral grounds useless and unnecessary surgery, that which is not required for either the physical or mental well-being of the patient. The principle is intuitively known and formulates in abstract language what nearly everyone knows by common sense. And even when it is not reflexly articulated, it is the practical norm which as a matter of fact guides all good surgical practice.

The principle of totality is a useful but limited principle. It explains why and when surgical mutilation or wounding is morally permissible. But it does not tell us anything about another question: when is surgery morally obligatory?

Obligatory and Optional Surgery

With the advancement of the science and art of medicine, many medical and surgical procedures are now regarded by the medical profession as routine and established practices. Therefore, medical personnel are often inclined to draw the moral conclusion that if these procedures are available they ought to be used. But that is not the way theological moralists reason. They attend closely to all the nonmedical human factors that bear on the situation before they draw any moral conclusions.

In this age of scientific medicine it will be instructive for us to consider the human wisdom of moralists of the past. Their humanity led them to appreciate that there are a great number of circumstances which would make efforts to stay alive only optional, not morally obligatory, even if these efforts were certain to be successful. Most of their examples are out of date, and their practical conclusions would no longer be valid today. But they illustrate for us their acute sensitivity to the human and morally relevant factors that should go into such a decision. In the age of technology such human considerations are too likely to be simply passed over.

The earlier moralists listed a number of nonmedical reasons that would justify a person's decision not to undergo surgery or medical treatment that would save his life. Gerald Kelly, S.J., gives the following examples: "Leaving home to go to a more healthful climate; the maiden's repugnance to being treated by a (male) physician or surgeon; the amputation of a limb; or other major operations, especially those involving the opening of the abdomen; and all very costly treatments."[5]

Those moralists, of course, were writing in a different context from today's. Leaving home no longer entails packing all one's belongings on a burro, facing the rigors of weather, mountains, desert, wild animals, and bandits, foraging for food along the way, and, after traveling in this way for a month or two, probably never seeing friends and family again.

A maiden who would find it repugnant to be treated by a male doctor would be rather rare today, but even if such a maiden could be found, a female doctor (and psychiatrist) could readily be provided for her. Thanks to modern anesthetics and disinfectants, amputations are no longer so horribly painful and so likely to prove lethal as they were in the past. And thanks to modern prosthetics and reconstructive surgery, an amputee does not have to look forward to a shameful, dependent, and useless life as a disfigured cripple. Moreover, while a major operation in the past usually was more dangerous to the patient than the disease or condition itself, the advent of modern surgery has meant that major operations usually do not involve excruciating pain or great risk to life.

Nonetheless, the important point is that theological moralists have always counted nonmedical human considerations as important factors in the determination of a person's moral obligation to save his life. The Lutheran moralist Helmut Thielicke expressed it this way: "If we speak about the duty of the doctor to preserve life, then not biological life as such is meant but *human* life. In order to characterize the life of man, other criteria are needed than those of the electrocardiograph and the electroencephalograph."[6]

Pope Pius XII summed up and adopted the traditional teaching of theological moralists. Avoiding their time-conditioned examples and practical casuistry, he formulated the humane principle that should guide man's practical decisions as he reasonably exercises his stewardship over his life: "Natural reason and Christian morals say that man has the right and the duty in case of serious illness to take the necessary treatment for the preservation of life and health. This duty that he has towards himself, towards God, towards the human community, and in most cases towards certain determined persons, derives from well-ordered charity, from submission to the Creator, from social justice, as well as from devotion towards his family. But normally, one is held to use only ordinary means—according to circumstances of persons, places, times, and culture—that is to say, means that do not involve any grave burden for oneself or another. A more strict obligation would be too burdensome for most men and would render the attainment of the higher, more important good too difficult. Life, death, all temporal activities are in fact subordinated to spiritual ends. On the other hand, one is not forbidden to take more than strictly necessary steps to preserve life and health, as long as one does not fail in some more serious duty."[7]

The principle, stated abstractly, is clear enough: proper and reasonable stewardship over our lives obliges us to make use of ordinary means to preserve them; we are permitted to use extraordinary means if we want to, but are under no obligation to do so.[8] The practical difficulty lies in determining in concrete circumstances what means are to be counted as ordinary and what measures should be judged extraordinary.

There is a special danger of confusion in the use of this terminology because the medical profession often uses the terms *ordinary* and *extraordinary* in a more restricted sense than moralists commonly do. Physicians usually define as ordinary means all established medical and surgical procedures appropriate to a given illness within the limits of availability. And they consider extraordinary means to be procedures which are incompletely established, frankly experimental, or bizarre.

Moralists, on the other hand, classify as ordinary means all medicines, treatments, and operations which offer a reasonable hope of benefit to the patient and which can be obtained and used without excessive expense, pain, or other inconvenience to the patient or others. The pope simply describes ordinary means as "means that do not involve any grave burden for oneself or another."

Specific means cannot be categorized as ordinary or extraordinary according to some mathematical formula. The question is determined according to the reasonable judgment of prudent and conscientious men. No permanent list of ordinary and extraordinary means can be drawn up because *ordinary* and *extraordinary* are relative terms. They are relative to the level and availability of medical technology and to the nonmedical human factors in a particular situation. What is ordinary and what is extraordinary can only be determined by a prudent judgment made, as the pope said, "according to circumstances of persons, places, times, and cultures." As an aid in making such situational judgments, it will be useful to consider some practical cases and to see how moralists generally evaluate them.

Some Contemporary Cases

Today, in those areas of the world where modern medicine is practiced, most surgical operations, even major operations, must be classified as ordinary means of preserving life. Appendectomies, gastric resections, hysterectomies, mastectomies, cholecystectomies, amputations, and so forth are, at least in normal circumstances, ordinary means and therefore morally obligatory. Although there is always some risk, pain, expense, or other inconvenience connected with such operations, none is usually so serious as to excuse a person from his obligation to preserve his life.

However, there are still operations that are so dangerous that they must be considered extraordinary means and therefore not morally mandatory but elective procedures. For instance, certain types of brain or heart surgery are extremely risky even when they are performed by competent surgeons supported by a good medical team. The surgical removal of a brain tumor is often highly dangerous. One estimate is that 10 to 20 percent of such surgery terminates fatally.[9] The risk in heart surgery varies with the nature of the operation. In general, about 97 percent of the patients who undergo open-heart surgery for rheumatic heart disease survive the operation, whereas an older but now outdated operation such as poudrage for coronary artery disease carried with it a mortality rate of about 10 percent.[10]

In each case of surgery the prognosis depends to a large degree on the nature of the operation, the age and general condition of the patient, the skill of the surgical team, the specific procedure used, and so on. The attending physician is best able to estimate the amount of risk involved in each instance.

Although no exact mathematical norm can be established, moralists generally estimate that if the mortality rate for a particular operation is around 10 to 15 percent, that operation should be classified as extraordinary means. And if the chances are more than one out of ten that a particular patient will not survive a certain operation because of his age or some other chronic condition, then that operation should be considered an extraordinary means for that patient. In such circumstances an individual may choose to take the chance and undergo surgery. Or he may choose to let the disease take its natural course rather than face the immediate risk of death in surgery.

In modern medical practice amputations are far less common than in the past, and prosthetic advances make a nearly normal life possible for most amputees. Still, there are situations in which the consequences of such an operation would be more than can be morally demanded. For instance, a diabetic old man whose life could be saved only by the amputation of his legs might reasonably prefer to die rather than to live out the rest of his life in bed.

A quadruple amputee in many instances faces a very difficult and humiliating life of almost total uselessness and dependency on others. It can be easily understood that some people would rather die than live out such a miserable life. Almost all moralists agree that one need not undergo such extreme physical mutilation even to preserve life.

Moralists would also understand the position of a Jehovah's Witness who, because of religious convictions, would not be willing to save his life by means of a blood transufsion. Blood transfusions today are surely an ordinary means of preserving life, but the great subjective repugnance of a Jehovah's Witness could make it an extraordinary means for him.[11]

The cost of the necessary medical and surgical treatment is also a factor in determining whether a treatment should be counted as ordinary or extraordinary means. If the expense involved in a certain treatment would cause grave hardship to an individual or his family, he may choose to forgo it. A man is required to use only ordinary means to preserve his life, and there are some amounts of money that would have to be counted as extraordinary.

It is no secret that surgical and medical costs are high. But we do not always realize how high they can get. The Gottschalk Committee estimated that the average cost of a kidney transplant is about $13,300.[12] In-center dialysis costs about $15,000 a year. Ten-year survival would thus cost a family $150,000. Home dialysis now costs about the same for the first year and $3,000 to $5,000 a year afterwards. To maintain an individual on home dialysis for ten years can cost as much as $65,000.

A newspaper account in the *Chicago Sun-Times* recently disclosed that Rev. and Mrs. George Depfer of Leesburg, Virginia, have had to pay close to $80,000 from family earnings over the past sixteen years for the necessary treatment of their son, who is a hemophiliac.[13] According to the National Hemophilia Foundation, Factor VIII (cryoprecipitate), which is used to restore the clotting factors to a hemophiliac's blood, costs between $10,000 and $22,000 for a year's supply, depending on the severity of the case. It could easily cost over a million dollars to keep a hemophiliac alive until the age of sixty.

In most Western nations insurance companies or the state pick up a large part of the bill in many cases. Generally speaking, an individual can secure the means necessary to preserve his life even though he cannot personally pay for them. But that is not always true. The problem of delivering the necessary health care to both the poor and the average man is still a critical one in the United States, and it is probably the most urgent medico-moral question facing us today. Until it is resolved we will continue to face situations in which individuals will not be able to obtain the care they need without incurring real financial hardship.

Treatments which are so costly as to place a grave financial burden on oneself or one's family are elective and not morally obligatory. As Paul Ramsey said: "The medical-moral imperative is not first to save life at these costs, and seek by some future course of action to remedy the human costs of warding off death. It works the other way around: the social distribution of medical care, removing or lessening these human costs, can alone transfer presently elective (because costly) procedures into imperative ones."[14]

Modern surgery and medical treatments very often involve some pain or discomfort. But anesthetics usually remove almost all the pain of an operation, and other sedatives keep the patient reasonably comfortable during the postoperative period. Therefore, the pain of an operation would make it an extraordinary means only in the most unusual circumstances.

Nevertheless, there are procedures that would leave the patient in permanent postoperative distress (through severe incapacitation or emotional embarrassment and shame), and those procedures would have to be judged extraordinary means. For instance, if a consequence of an otherwise successful surgery will be some severe and relatively permanent hardship for an individual, that surgery is optional but not morally required. Similarly, six months or a year in bed or in an iron lung could constitute so grave a burden for an individual that such treatment would have to be classified as extraordinary means to preserve his life.[15]

A person may desire to use every available means to stay alive, but there are limits to what he or she is morally obliged to do. One is morally obliged only to use ordinary means, those which do not carry with them any grave burden for oneself or others. Paul Ramsey once suggested that a sign be posted over all operating rooms saying: "Choose all you who enter here! You *must* choose before entering here and you *may* choose not to enter here."[16]

Letting Some Babies Die

Normally the patient himself should make the choice of using or forgoing extraordinary means. It is his decision, and whenever possible the physician should follow the wishes of his patient.

But sometimes the patient will not be able to make the decision for himself; someone else will have to make it for him. An obvious instance is the case of a small child or infant. Ordinarily parents must make the decision for their children. In such cases the parents are bound by the same moral obligations as the child: they must use ordinary means to preserve life, and they may, but need not, use extraordinary means.

However, it is one thing to know the principle that we are obliged to use ordinary but not extraordinary means; it is quite another to face the difficult choice between using or not using the extraordinary and therefore elective means. As a practical guideline the principle is severely limited. Knowledge of the abstract principle will not substitute for the ambiguous and agonizing practical decision that has to be made.

Usually parents will want everything possible done to save their child. But what if the measures that must be taken to preserve the life of a baby will bankrupt the family? What if the costs will be so great that the other children, as well as the parents, will suffer grave and permanent hardship? What if there is no assurance that the extraordinary measures will be successful? What would the baby want done if he were old enough to make the decision for himself?

These are the kinds of questions that parents must face as they try to decide whether or not to authorize the use of extraordinary means to save the life of a child. They must try to weigh all the values involved and choose in favor of what seems best for everyone concerned.

Probably the most difficult decisions that parents have to make concern babies who are born deformed. We have already described the case of a spina bifida with a meningomyelocele.[17] Similar cases are not uncommon in our hospitals today.

The medical profession seems to be sharply divided on what should or should not be done for grossly malformed infants. Many doctors have simply withdrawn lifesaving measures from grossly malformed infants, allowing them quietly to die, and telling the parents that their babies were stillborn. Other doctors feel that they must do everything in their power to preserve life, arguing that a condition that is incurable today may be curable tomorrow.

The courts have provided little guidance in this area. Judges have countermanded the decisions of parents and ordered that necessary blood transfusions be given or surgery performed to save the lives of older children. But until recently the courts have taken no legal action against parents or physicians who have decided to withhold necessary treatment from grossly malformed infants.

The first legal decision in this area was made in February 1974 by Maine's Superior Court Judge David G. Roberts, who ruled: "At the moment of live birth there does exist a human being entitled to the fullest protection of the law. The most basic right enjoyed by every human being is the right to life itself."[18]

The case concerned Baby Boy Houle, who was born with his entire left side malformed. He had no left eye, practically no left ear, a number of unfused vertebrae, and a tracheoesophageal fistula. He developed pneumonia, and because of either lung or heart abnormalities, his brain was damaged by lack of oxygen. Also, his reflexes deteriorated, his natural breathing periodically stopped, and he developed convulsive seizures. The medical prognosis was that a gastrotomy probably would save his life, but that he would be palsied, blind, deaf, unable to communicate, and probably unable to stand.

The baby's father, Sgt. Robert H. T. Houle, instructed the doctors not to perform the gastrotomy and to discontinue the intravenous feeding that was keeping the baby alive. The doctor and the hospital did not want to take the responsibility for carrying out Sergeant Houle's wishes, and so they took the case to Judge Roberts for a ruling and received the decision to operate. The operation was successfully performed. Nonetheless, two days later Baby Boy Houle died.[19]

In the *New England Journal of Medicine,* Drs. Raymond Duff and A. G. M. Campbell reported the results of a study of 299 deaths among 2,171 children treated in the special-care nursery at Yale-New Haven Hospital over a 2½-year period. In 43 instances the parents and doctor jointly decided not to treat the infant and to let it die. The other 256 babies were given the best treatment that modern medicine can provide, but few of these survived any longer than those who were untreated. Those who did survive longer were often kept alive in a pathetic condition. One infant was kept breathing for five months on a mechanical respirator.[20]

The question of what should or should not be done to save grossly malformed infants has never been thoroughly discussed, let alone settled, by either the medical profession or the courts. Neither have theological moralists as yet subjected the question to any thorough ethical analysis and debate. Perhaps the reason for this apparent lack of interest in the question is that in the past most grossly malformed infants did not survive for very long no matter what was done for them. The problem was not as urgent as it is today, now that an increasing number of such babies can be saved from death, but at the cost of disablement and retardation.

A few of the earlier moralists have touched on the question, but only in a very fleeting way. Charles McFadden once expressed the opinion that a monstrosity must be placed in a heating bassinet. He argued that a heating bassinet is an ordinary means of sustaining infant life and that therefore its use is obligatory even for monstrosities. At the same time he judged that it would be extraordinary means and therefore not obligatory to have an artificial esophagus made for a baby with congenital atresia.[21]

In an article published in 1950, Gerald Kelly reported McFadden's opinions without comment.[22] However, he indicated in a footnote that he was in agreement with McFadden's fundamental principle—that "the determination of ordinary and extraordinary [means should] begin with the mentally normal."[23]

Paul Ramsey has indicated his disagreement with McFadden and Kelly: "Since we ought not to absolutize the distinction between 'usual' and 'heroic' treatment of newborn babies, not to place 'a monstrosity in a heating bassinet' or to stop opposing the infection to which it is prone cannot be declared morally wrong while an operation is said to be optional to provide a child who was born with congenital atresia with an artificial or implanted esophagus."

Ramsey explains his reason in this way: "'Ordinary' or imperative and 'extraordinary' or only elective treatments are . . . not fixed categories. The feeling that infants should be given the greatest protection does not alone settle what we ought to do. Life in the first of it and life in the last of it are both prismatic cases of human helplessness. The question is, What does loyalty to the newborn and to the dying require of us? Consistently, we could say that both should unqualifiedly be given every effort that might save or prolong their existence. But if a balancing judgment is permitted—even morally mandatory—concerning whether proposed remedies will be beneficial to the adult dying, the same reasoning cannot be preemptorially excluded from our care of the newborn. If in the case of terminal patients the quality of life they can expect enters into the determination of whether even ordinary or customary measures would be beneficial and should or should not be used, cannot the same be said of infants? It is not obvious that an anecephaletic baby should be respirated while a grown man in prolonged coma should no longer be helped to breathe."[24]

Writing in the medical context of 1956, Edwin Healy,

S.J., gives his opinion on three pertinent cases.[25] The first concerns a baby born with a single head and two bodies. A very delicate throat operation costing several thousand dollars would be necessary to keep the baby alive. Healy's solution is that because of the very heavy financial burden that would be placed on the family, the operation would be extraordinary means and therefore elective but not obligatory.

The second case is that of an infant who can neither suck nor swallow, so that he must be fed through a stomach tube. Gavage will be permanently necessary if he is to be kept alive. Moreover, there are indications that he may be an imbecile. Healy argues that the fact that the child is probably an imbecile is an irrelevant consideration, since every infant, whether normal or abnormal, must be given the benefit of ordinary means to preserve life. However, in this instance he thinks that the necessity of providing gavage over a long period of time, i.e., six months or more, would be so burdensome to the parents that it would be extraordinary means and therefore not obligatory.

The third case concerns an infant born with a hydrocephalic condition. If it lives, it will never be normal and will be a very grave burden to the parents. To keep it alive artificial respiration is required immediately. Healy argues that the physician must use artificial respiration to save the infant: "Artificial respiration of a temporary nature is an ordinary means of tiding a person over a crisis, and therefore it is obligatory. The fact that this young patient is horribly abnormal does not alter the solution of the case. Every infant, no matter how grossly deformed he may be, is a human being and as such has the same right to life as that which is enjoyed by a perfectly normal child. Whatever a physician would be obliged to do for a normal child, he must do for this hydrocephalic."

In a recent landmark article published simultaneously

in the *Journal of the American Medical Association* and *America,* Richard McCormick expresses his disagreement with the earlier Catholic moralists. He argues that the quality of the life to be lived is a relevant consideration in the determination of whether or not a life ought to be saved. As a practical guideline he suggests that if the infant's "potential for human relationship" is "simply non-existent or would be utterly submerged in the mere struggle to survive, that life has achieved its potential." The capacity to relate cannot be determined by a mathematical formula, and the decision to let a baby die or to save it will remain the burden of parents in consultation with doctors. In many cases the judgment will be ambiguous and unclear. But in some cases it will be relatively easy. For instance, there is little doubt that the anecephalic infant is without relational potential, whereas the same is not true of the mongloloid. Father McCormick argues: "It is neither in-human nor unchristian to say that there comes a point where an individual's condition itself represents the negation of any truly human—i.e., relational—potential. When that point is reached, is not the best treatment no treatment?"[26]

The foregoing examples represent the present state of the discussion of this unpleasant problem in the ethical literature. It is evident that a more thorough discussion is still necessary. Because the problem is presenting itself with increasing frequency and is coming to the attention of the courts and the media, such a discussion is bound to come. In the meantime, I would like to offer the following opinions.

It seems that in the great majority of cases of grossly malformed infants, the means necessary to save life must be classified as extraordinary means and therefore elective, not mandatory. The reason is that, very frequently, the means necessary to preserve life either will impose a grave hardship on the infant or the family or will fail to confer any significant benefit on the infant. No one is obliged to do what is practically useless. In very many instances there are no measures that will keep the seriously deformed infant alive for very long. Even in the presence of the best care that modern medicine can provide, such infants are already in the grip of an irreversible process of dying, and even measures generally considered ordinary would be useless. They would not confer any significant benefit on the dying infant and therefore would not be morally obligatory.

The more difficult cases will be those in which a grossly malformed baby will be able to survive for a long time if usual and convenient measures are employed, for instance, artificial respiration for a short time or some simple and routine surgical operation. Most of the theologians who touched on this question in the past felt that the deformity of the baby was an irrelevant consideration. They held that if a certain treatment was regarded as ordinary means for a normal child, it would also be ordinary and mandatory for a grossly deformed child. Healy's argument was that "every infant, no matter how grossly deformed he may be, is a human being and as such has the same right to life as that which is enjoyed by a perfectly normal child."[27]

But notice that Healy has subtly switched the question on us. He argues that a deformed child has the same right to life as a normal one. But the question under discussion does not concern one's right to live. It concerns one's duty or moral obligation to live—and that is entirely another matter.

Everyone has a right to use extraordinary means to stay alive. If a man wants to use extraordinary means, he has a right to say so, and, whenever possible, the doctor must comply with his wishes. But the whole point of the issue is that one does not have the duty to use extraordinary means. Morally these means are elective, not mandatory.

If an operation or treatment will cause serious hardship to oneself or others, one need not submit to it. Healy considers this case: "Thomas, a forty-year-old man, is deformed and badly crippled. For many years he has been a grave burden to his wife; and he well realizes that the required surgery, by saving his life, will increase his wife's hardships and exact even greater sacrifices on her part in the future." Healy's solution: "Thomas . . . has no obligation to submit to the surgery." In fact, he goes on to say that charity probably would oblige him to forgo the live-saving operation.[28]

The only important difference between a deformed and badly crippled forty-year-old man like Thomas and a grossly deformed infant is that Thomas can decide for himself whether he will use the necessary means to stay alive, whereas someone else, generally the parents, must make the decision for the infant. Moralists have always recognized the right and duty of parents to make crucial decisions for their children. They must make these decisions in terms of the child's good. They must interpret, as it were, the child's reasonable wishes. And they cannot presume that a grossly deformed child would reasonably desire to cling to a deformed, crippled, or monstrous existence, no matter what hardships this prolonged existence would cause the child or the family.

We must be extremely cautious here. We do not want to set ourselves on the slippery slope to Dachau, where some men made decisions for others about whether or not their lives were worth living. Parents should make their decision in the child's interests, trying to determine what such a deformed infant would reasonably want. Therefore, although moral generalizations are very difficult, some objective standard or guideline seems to be called for. I think that the practical guideline suggested by McCormick is very useful here. Does the infant have the potential for human relationship; does he at least have the capacity to relate to other human beings?

This does not supply us with a precise formula for making all the necessary decisions in this area. But at least it gives us a practical, objective standard which will help to illumine many cases and guard against excesses. As McCormick has pointed out, there is little doubt that the anecephalic infant is without relational potential, whereas the same is not true of the mongloloid. Unclear and ambiguous cases will still remain. But the fact of twilight does not mean that we cannot tell the difference between day and night.

We must remember also that *ordinary* and *extraordinary means* are not fixed categories. They are relative to every situation. What would be a light and bearable burden to one family might be intolerable to another. To help parents make the decision for their deformed child doctors should meet with them as soon as possible after delivery. They should explain as accurately as possible the infant's problem, the measures necessary to save it, and the kind of life that these measures might succeed in preserving. It seems that in many cases the parents may licitly decide to give the infant only normal nourishment and thus to let it die.

Paul Ramsey once wisely observed: "In the first of life, a human being may be seized by his own unique dying. Indeed, far from taking the death of the aged and the enormous death rate of zygotes and miscarriages to be a part of the problem of evil, a religious man is likely to take this as a sign that the Lord of life has beset us behind and before in this dying life we are called to live and celebrate. There is an acceptable death of the life of all flesh no less in the first than in the last of it. An ethical man may always gird himself to oppose this enemy, but not the religious ethical man."[29]

CHAPTER **2**

ORGAN TRANSPLANTATION

Homografts for human beings began in 1920 with skin transplants between identical twins. In 1951 Dr. David Hume of Boston used a cadaver organ to perform the first kidney transplant on a human being. And in 1954 Dr. Hume's colleagues, Dr. Joseph E. Murray and Dr. John Merrill, performed the first human kidney transplant from a living donor, using identical twins.

Although Richard Herrick, who received this transplant from his twin brother, survived for eight years after the operation, most of the kidney transplants that were performed during the 1950s were unsuccessful because the transplanted organ was not assimilated by the recipient body. The research of Professor Peter Medawar and his colleagues revealed that the human body possesses an active immunization mechanism which destroys or rejects foreign tissue. Continued experiments, however, showed that this is not an insurmountable obstacle to organ transplantation. The development of strong immunosuppressive drugs like azathioprine (in 1961) made the transplantation of human organs considerably more practicable.

Today most organ transplantation must still be described

as highly experimental. This is certainly true of the transplantation of hearts, lungs, liver, and spleen. But even though the rate of failure is still high in kidney transplantation, it can now be regarded as therapeutic rather than experimental surgery. With the perfection of immunosuppressive therapy we can reasonably expect that in the future every form of organ transplantation will pass from the category of experimental to that of therapeutic medicine.

There are special moral issues connected with experimental surgery, as we shall see in the next chapter. But these are not the only moral issues that arise. If we disregard for the moment the experimental nature of most types of organ transplantation, we can consider the basic moral problem which is involved in any organ transplantation, no matter how safe and secure it may be.

Primum non nocere is an elementary medical principle which has always been recognized by doctors. In fact, physicians generally have been more sensitive than moralists to the importance of the integrity of the flesh. Philosophers and theologians are inclined to spiritualize man into some being other than what he is. But physicians and surgeons more readily recognize man as the body of his soul as well as the soul of his body. They are not as easily duped by the Cartesian dualism of mind and body as the rest of Western society. Their work is with embodied life, and they know from long experience that physical wholeness in man is intimately associated with psychological and spiritual health. Therefore, they are always reluctant to destroy healthy human tissue.

Nevertheless, the destruction of healthy tissue is sometimes necessary. It is necessary to protect the life or health of an individual—for instance, to prevent the spread of cancer—or to protect the life of another—for instance, to save a fetus. Further, because cadaver organs are in short supply and because the success rate is higher when a living related donor is used, it may also be necessary to remove healthy tissue from one human being in order to save the life of another.

However, because a thing is necessary or useful, it does not automatically follow that it is therefore morally good or permissible. If our behavior is to be truly human, we must also have an ethic of means. At this moment in history there is little likelihood that our thinking about organ transplantation will be influenced by the totalitarian view of man which governed medical practice in Nazi Germany. But there is some danger that it will be influenced by the technological, mechanistic, "spare parts" mentality of the present.

We are not merely parts of each other any more than we are parts of society. The good of the individual is not identified with or subordinated to the good of society or the good of other men. Each person has a finality of his own. He is not a means but an end in himself. No one therefore may be forced to give a part of his body to someone else. That is why the free and informed consent of the living donor is always essential.

Obtaining such consent, however, involves a number of subtle problems. Informed consent implies that the donor is made aware of the risk he is taking. The physical risks assumed in giving a kidney are not enormous, but they are real. The human body can function adequately on one healthy kidney. But if that kidney becomes diseased in the future, the donor himself becomes a transplant candidate. One estimate calculates that the risk in giving a kidney is equivalent to the risk involved in driving a car 8,000 miles a year.[1] Another estimate is that there is a 1 out of 2,000 chance that the donor will die during the operation and 1 out of 1,500 chance that his life will be endangered afterwards.[2] Such risks may reasonably be undertaken. But there are risks, and the donor must freely decide to accept them.

Another problem is obtaining consent which is truly free.

Usually the living donor is a member of the immediate family. Unrelated persons who offer a kidney for transplantation are very often psychoneurotics who should not be used. In fact, some transplant centers will not use an unrelated living donor under any circumstances. Normally a transplant operation is performed either from a living related donor or from an unrelated cadaver. From a strictly medical point of view, a living donor is preferred, since the chance of success with a living related donor is considerably higher. This creates a special problem, for there is considerable risk that the "free consent" of the relative may not be as free as it may seem.

Genuine love often prompts a relative to sacrifice an organ to save the life of a member of his family. This is frequently true of parents regarding their children. But there is often considerably more reluctance on the part of sons and daughters to the idea of sacrificing an organ for their parents or for their brothers or sisters.

The love that prompts a person to give up an organ for a relative must be admired, but it cannot be coerced. The fundamental moral imperative is that no organ may be taken from anyone without his free, informed consent.

There is always danger that a relative will feel heavy psychological pressure to give a needed kidney to another member of the family. Family members can subtly or overtly exert enormous pressure on a relative to "volunteer," and if he should refuse he might have to live with immense guilt or under lifelong censure. Because of the common danger of this kind of family blackmail, physicians should be very cautious about accepting the organ of a living related donor. Every precaution should be taken to guarantee the freedom of the donor's decision.

Dr. Henry K. Beecher reports a typical practice of transplant surgeons: "The donor is told that if he does not want to give a kidney no one will know, for the physician will state that the donor is unsuitable. In these circumstances about three of five donors are found to be genuine volunteers."[3]

The fact that 40 percent of the volunteers were not truly free indicates that the physician should be extremely careful in assessing the freedom of anyone's consent. Some people will feel so pressured inwardly by the prospect of guilt that they will never outwardly admit their unwillingness. If he detects such covert unwillingness, the physician should simply reject the donor on "medical grounds," without revealing the real reason to him or anyone else.

The ethical problem is even more difficult when the donor is a child. Legally, minor children are permitted to be used as donors only with the written permission of their parents or guardians. But that legal fact does not resolve all the moral problems.

Very young children are incapable of giving informed consent. Parents must "interpret" their will and give consent in their name. There obviously are grave dangers involved whenever one person gives such consent for someone else. Some of the dangers here are that the parents will tend to make their decision with a controlling bias towards the needs of the sick child or that, in the case of twins, parents will succumb to the subtle temptation to think of the two as a single being rather than as unique, autonomous, and separate individuals. Because children can be so easily manipulated into thinking that they must give up an organ to save the life of a brother or sister, some physicians think that the law should take the decision out of anyone's hands and prohibit the giving of an organ by anyone under seventeen or eighteen years old.[4]

The Theoretical Problem

The free, informed consent of the donor is imperative. But it alone does not settle the issue. It may come as a surprise to some that, even assuming the fully free consent of the donor, moral theologians have had difficulty in justifying organ transplantation.

The act of voluntarily giving an organ to save the life of another may be motivated by selfless love, but medical ethics is not solely or even primarily an ethics of inner motive. The mere presence of love as a motivating factor does not settle every issue. What we are doing is equally as important as why we are doing it.

The development of organ transplantation as a medical possibility during the 1950s posed a new problem for moralists. For the first time in the history of medicine, a surgical procedure was adopted in which a perfectly healthy person was permanently injured in order to improve the well-being of another. A question arose about the limits imposed by man's proper stewardship over his body and life: Do we have the right to permit ourselves to be damaged in our bodily integrity even if our motive is altruistic love?

Before the transplantation of organs had been envisioned, moralists had worked out the theoretical principle—the principle of totality—that justified the mutilation or destruction of members or organs of the human body: Since the parts of the body exist for the good of the whole, they may be sacrificed for the good of the whole. In other words, parts of a man's body may be damaged or destroyed when such an act is necessary for his own good.

It was obvious that the principle of totality did not cover the new procedure of organ transplantation. So the question came up for debate: Do the parts of the human body exist exclusively for the good of the individual or do they also have a wider finality? This question had a particular importance for Catholic moralists writing in the 1950s, because some believed that papal declarations had settled the issue.

In his encyclical on Christian marriage, *Casti Connubii,*

issued in 1930, Pope Pius XI had said: "Private individuals have no other power over members of their bodies than that which pertains to their natural ends; and they are not free to destroy or mutilate or in any other way render themselves unfit for their natural functions, except when no other provision can be made for the good of the whole body."[5] And in 1952 his successor, Pope Pius XII, had said: "Each of the members, for example, the hand, the foot, the heart, the eye, is an integral part destined by all its being to be inserted in the whole organism. Outside the organism it has not, by its very nature, any sense, any finality. It is wholly absorbed by the totality of the organism to which it is attached."[6]

After lengthy debate most Catholic theologians concluded that papal teaching did not in fact prohibit organ transplantation. In *Casti Connubii* Pope Pius XI was mainly concerned with condemning eugenic sterilization. He was not professedly discussing the general problem of mutilation. Much less was he trying to settle the question of organ transplantation, a question which did not arise until more than twenty years after he was writing.

Pope Pius XII's statement was made about two years before the first successful kidney transplant from a living donor. Debates on the topic already were going on in the moral literature, and no doubt the pope was aware of them. If he had wanted to address the issue, he had ample opportunity to do so in his numerous addresses on medico-moral problems. But he never did.

His strong statement that a member of the human body has no finality outside it must be interpreted in its context. Its context is not a discussion of the new medical procedure of transplanting organs. Rather it is an attack on the totalitarian concept of society and the Nazi abuses in human experimentation. The thrust of the pope's argument was that the members of a society are persons with a meaning and finality of their own, one which transcends that of the society to which they belong, whereas the members of the human body have no meaning or finality outside it. Theologians argue that the pope did not have the question of transplants in mind and that his statement has no application to that problem.[7]

This exegesis became the more commonly accepted interpretation among Catholic theologians, and it provoked no opposition from the Holy See. Thus a common consensus developed in the Catholic theological community: supposing the free and informed consent of the living donor, organ transplantation is morally permissible provided that it confers a proportionate benefit on the recipient and does not expose the donor to great risk of life or does not deprive him completely of some important function.

The principle justifying organ transplantation therefore is not the principle of totality.[8] The principle of totality provides a useful rationale for surgery in general, but it is limited in its intent and range of application. It neither allows nor prohibits organ transplantation. It asserts that the members of the body are for the good of the whole body without denying that they also can have another finality.

The principle which justifies the sacrifice of an organ for the good of another person is the law of fraternal charity. There is no subordination existing between any one person and others, but there is an ordination, an ordering of one to another. The unity among men makes our neighbor "another self," so that we may do for him what we may do for ourselves.

The principle of totality is a useful rule, for it reminds us that we are our bodies. It prevents us from depreciating the importance of embodied life and existence in the flesh. But it is the law of fraternal charity which tells us of our call to give ourselves in love to others in need. Without it, the principle of totality could become a mask for egocentric self-preservation.

The Cadaver Donor

Some transplant centers do not encourage the use of living donors at all. Others frequently cannot find a medically suitable living donor. The obvious alternative is a cadaver donor. But these too are frequently in short supply. Most of the organs needed to save human lives are not transplanted. They are buried or burned.

Some resistance to the use of cadavers for organ transplantation derives from superstitious religious beliefs. Some people oppose the use of their organs for transplants because of an exaggerated reverence for the sacredness of the body or because of an excessively physicalist understanding of the Christian doctrine of resurrection. They do not want to "desecrate" after death bodies that were temples of God during life. Or they do not want to rise from their graves on the last day and find that they have no lungs, kidneys, or heart.

Resistance also comes from some funeral directors who feel a threat to their business. Neat embalming is difficult if an organ has been removed, and especially so if several are gone. It is even worse for morticians if the whole body is willed to medical research. One funeral director put it plainly: "With no body, there is no funeral. If there are no funerals, there are no funeral directors."[9]

Most people have no objection to the use of their organs for transplants after death. According to a 1968 Gallup poll, 70 percent of American adults said they were willing to donate an organ after death. Very few, however, make the necessary arrangements. The result is that their organs are buried with them.

One proposal has been for a general law allowing the routine salvaging of human organs for transplantation after death. According to this plan everyone would be presumed at law to be a cadaver donor. Anyone who objected on any grounds could simply let his objection be known before death, and his wishes would be respected when he died. But if one did not object during life, his organs could be salvaged after death if they were suitable and necessary for a transplant.

A different proposal was, in fact, enacted into law in 1968 and is now in effect in all of the fifty states. The Uniform Anatomical Gift Act affirms the right of anyone over eighteen years old and mentally competent to donate his organs for transplantation after death, and it denies the right of any relative to override the decision of the donor.

At least in theory the Uniform Anatomical Gift Act is preferable to the proposal for the routine salvaging of human organs. By making the retrieval of organs automatic except in the face of expressed refusal, the proposal relies on inaction rather than action. Given normal human inertia this would certainly seem to be the more effective way of insuring the needed supply of organs for transplants. But the truth is that if this proposal were enacted into law, most people would not be real donors at all. The urgent need for human organs would better be met. But it would be met not by personal giving but by societal taking.

The effective supply of medically necessary spare parts, important as it is, is not the only human or moral concern here. As Paul Ramsey sensitively observed: "The positive consent called for by Gift Acts, answering the need for gifts by encouraging real givers, meets the measure of authentic community among men. The routine taking of organs would deprive individuals of the exercise of the virtue of generosity. If, as it is said, the young rarely think about their own deaths or about giving their organs upon death, then they should be constrained and enabled to do so by the institutions and practices of the laws we enact. . . . The moral sequels that might flow from education and action in line with the proposed Gift Acts may be of far more importance than prolonging lives routinely. The moral history of mankind is of more importance than its medical advancement, unless the latter can be joined with the former in a community of affirmative consent."[10]

The common objection to this position is that it is too idealistic and will not in fact insure that we obtain the organs we need. At least this much must be admitted: if the policy adopted in the Uniform Anatomical Gift Act is to remain morally defensible, it must be accompanied by widespread publicity and strong encouragement among the young people in our society. Needless to say, clergy and medical personnel share in this important responsibility.

Defining Death

Not very long ago medical textbooks were recommending that physicians place a mirror or feather in front of the nose to determine the occurrence of death. Cessation of respiration and heartbeat were the commonly accepted signs of death. Modern resuscitative techniques have made these ancient criteria inadequate.

What is more, transplant surgeons need a more exact definition of death. The transplantation of a kidney or a heart from a cadaver is technically possible as long as the organ has not deteriorated. It is morally imperative that a heart donor be dead. But it is medically imperative that he not be so dead that his heart cannot be used for a transplant.

There is, of course, only one reason why a person should be declared dead. A person should be declared dead because he is no longer alive, not because his organs are needed in order to keep someone else alive. But the possibility of organ transplantation makes it urgent for us to know in a particular instance whether a man is still a living patient or, in effect, an unburied corpse whose bodily functions of respiration and heartbeat are being artificially maintained.

Pope Pius XII said that the definition of death is a scientific rather than moral or religious problem, and that the resolution of the issue therefore lies outside the competence of the Church. In an address called "The Prolongation of Life," he declared: "It is in the physician's domain . . . to give a clear and precise definition of 'death' and of the 'moment of death' of a patient who dies without regaining consciousness. . . . As to the pronouncement of death in certain particular cases, the answer cannot be inferred from religious and moral principles, and consequently, it is an aspect lying outside the competence of the Church."[11]

As we shall presently see, this does not imply that there is no philosophical or human dimension to the question or that there are no ethical issues involved. It means that the establishment of criteria for ascertaining when death has occurred is a scientific, medical task.

From a medical standpoint death is a process that can be traced through four stages—clinical death, brain death, biological death, and cellular death.[12] Clinical death occurs when respiration and heartbeat stop. Sometimes clinical death can be reversed through resuscitative measures like artificial respiration and heart massage, and sometimes it cannot. Under normal temperatures the brain usually is damaged if it is deprived of oxygen for about ten minutes. Hence if clinical death is reversed by resuscitative measures, permanent brain damage may have resulted.

Brain death is the second stage in the dying process, and the brain itself dies in progressive stages. Clinical death is followed by death of the cortex, then death of the midbrain or diencephalon, and finally death of the brainstem. The higher levels of the brain control man's conscious existence. The lower levels control his nervous system and cardio-respiratory functions. Hence injury to the cortex can result in irreversible coma but not necessarily in irreversible brain death. It is therefore possible for a man to lie unconscious over many years without suffering cardiac or respiratory arrest.

Complete brain death results in biological death: all bodily life ceases. The ultimate result is cellular death. Some cells die more rapidly than others; for instance, hair and fingernails still grow for a short time after the death of the rest of the body.

That is the phenomenology of death. It is based on empirical observation. All scientists agree that it is an accurate description of the dying process.

But all do not agree on the set of medical criteria that should be used to determine when a man should be declared dead. Paul Ramsey has distinguished three schools of thought.[13] The first, he says, has not been endorsed by any responsible committee or organization, but it does exist in the popular mind and in the minds of some physicians. According to this view, human death means brain death, and the test for determining it is exclusively, or almost exclusively, the electroencephalograph, which records the electric impulses or waves in the brain. A flat or isoelectric EEG demonstrates that the person is dead. In this understanding Sen. Robert F. Kennedy was dead at 6:30 P.M. on 5 June 1968. For it was at that time, according to Dr. James Poppen, that his electric brain waves finally stopped, although his heart still continued to beat.

A second position also identifies human death with brain death. But it includes other testing procedures as well as the use of the electroencephalograph. The Declaration of the World Medical Association states: "The point of death of the different cells and organs is not so important as the certainty that the process has become irreversible by whatever techniques of resuscitation that may be employed. This determination will be based on clinical judgment supplemented if necessary by a number of diagnostic aids of which the electroencephalograph is currently the most helpful. However, no single technological criterion is entirely satisfactory in the present state of medicine nor can any one technological procedure be substituted for the overall judgment of the physician."[14]

Similarly, an ad hoc committee of the Harvard Medical School under the chairmanship of Dr. Henry K. Beecher has said that death is signified by a permanently nonfunctioning brain. This condition, the committee noted, can be satisfactorily diagnosed by (1) unreceptivity and unresponsitivity, (2) absence of movement or breathing, and (3) absence of reflexes. In addition, the committee observed, "of great confirmatory value is the flat or isoelectric EEG."[15]

If it is available, a properly functioning electroencephalograph in the hands of competent personnel is a useful instrument for confirming a diagnosis that irreversible brain death has occurred. But it is neither necessary nor sufficient in itself. Brain death, according to the Harvard committee, can be determined by a physician by means of the three clinical signs outlined above or "by the absence of circulation as judged by standstill of blood in the retinal vessels, or by the absence of cardiac activity." Death should be certified by two physicians, and before it is declared all of the tests should be repeated twenty-four hours later and should show no change. Also, when the tests are made, the patient's temperature should not be under 90° F (32.2° C.), nor should he be under the influence of central nervous depressants. Finally, the committee says that, as a precaution against ambiguity or legal problems, if brain death is diagnosed, the respirator should not be turned off and then death declared. Rather death should first be declared by the physician in charge, and only after the declaration of death should the artificial respirator be shut off.

The third position is the most traditional. Unlike the first two, it does not define death as brain death but as "the cessation of *integrated* life functions."[16] In this view death does not consist simply in the death of the brain any more than it consists in the cessation of heartbeat or respiration.

Death is not decided by the failure of one or two organs; it is decided by the integrated failure of the structural parts and the central nervous system. This means that death is what it has always been—the permanent cessation of all heart, lung, and brain activity. According to this position, it is not so much the definition of death as the clinical tests for determining it that need updating and refinement.

The foregoing is, I believe, a fairly accurate summary of the current literature on updating death. I also believe that there is no important practical difference of opinion among those writing on the subject. The first position, which defines death as brain death and requires only the use of the EEG to determine it, can simply be dismissed. As Ramsey points out, it has never been endorsed by any responsible committee studying the question, and it exists only in the public mind and in the minds of a few physicians. It represents only a popular misconception of what the current discussion is about.

Concerning the second and third positions, Paul Ramsey has wisely observed: "There is not so much difference between [them], if we remember that doctors are not theoreticians debating the meaning of death but practical men primarily concerned to establish agreed-upon procedures for stating that death has occurred. Various sets of criteria are currently being proposed by committees of physicians. The discussion focuses on the procedures for determining that a man has died. Physicians can afford to be nominalists about the meaning of death except as this is a function of the procedural question. While among them as well as the public at large there is a good deal of talk about brain death, it is safe to say that for the medical profession death operationally means what is stated by the use of sound and sufficient criteria for telling when a man has died. These are almost always manifold tests or procedures, not solely brain tests, if by the latter EEG is meant. . . . We should therefore take the current discussions of death to be practical proposals for revising the procedures for stating that death has occurred, and not as discussions of the theoretical meaning of death. So understood, I am emboldened to suggest that the various accounts of how death might better be reckoned are not proposing anything very startling."[17]

Roberta Simmons and Julie Fulton support Ramsey's reading of the debate: "Essentially the issue is not so much one of when a death has occurred as much as it is one of which criteria to use in determining it. In other words, most physicians feel fully capable of being able to diagnose brain death and of being able to decide when a patient is dead. But because they are anxious to avoid criticism, they feel bound—in the face of so much publicity about the issue—to utilize one set of criteria or another so as to be able to point to some objective sign of death."[18]

Prof. Paul Freund once remarked that the report of the ad hoc committee of the Harvard Medical School seemed to be "a set of guidelines on how to use a respirator."[19] Freund's remark is not as flippant as it might appear. For it points to the real issue underlying all of the recent discussion on updating death.

The immediate effect of brain death is the loss of capacity for spontaneous breathing. This in turn results in the stopping of the heart. But if the operation of the lungs is maintained by a respirator, the heart will continue to beat even though the brain is dead and there is no capability of spontaneous breathing. Therefore, the crucial practical question revolves around the patient whose brain is dead but whose heart still beats only because his lung life is being artificially maintained by a respirator. Is he to be counted as a living man or as an unburied corpse?

The thrust of all the recent medical literature is to say that he is an unburied corpse. Whether one locates death in the death of the brain or in the integrated failure of the brain, lungs, and heart, the practical conclusion is the same. A flat EEG is not in itself the decisive element. No one is to be declared dead who still has the potency of spontaneous respiration. But one who has no hope of ever recovering the power of spontaneous respiration because of irreversible destruction of the brain is no longer a living being, even though his heart and lung functions are being mechanically maintained.

From ancient times down to the recent past the cessation of breathing and heartbeat have been the accepted signs of death. Since the brain dies within a few minutes after breathing and heartbeat stop, these clinical signs formed an adequate criterion of death for physicians. They also were the norm at law. In *Thomas* vs. *Anderson* the California District Court of Appeal in 1950 simply quoted the definition of death from Black's *Law Dictionary* and concluded: "Death . . . does not occur until the heart stops beating and respiration ends."[20]

What the current literature on updating death is saying, in one way or another, is that this ancient criterion of death is not valid when modern resuscitative and supportive measures are used, because today mechanical and electrical instruments can produce respiration and heartbeat in a corpse.

The Harvard Medical School report suggests a reform in the current, but antiquated, legal concept of death. For this reform to occur, it suggests, "no statutory change in the law should be necessary since the law treats this question essentially as one of fact to be determined by physicians."[21]

It appears that such a reform is already under way. In May 1974 California Supreme Court Judge William J. Hayes ruled that "a person may be pronounced dead if, based on the usual and customary standards of medical practice, it is determined that the person has suffered irreversible cessation of brain function."[22]

Hayes' ruling was made in a charge to the jury in the murder trial of Andrew D. Lyons, who was accused of murdering Samuel M. Allen on 10 September 1973. Lyons' lawyer had argued that Allen did not die because Lyons shot him in the head on September 10, but because surgeons removed his heart for a transplant operation on September 12. Doctors had testified that all of Allen's brain activity had stopped shortly after he was shot, but that his heart had been kept functioning for two more days. The implication of Judge Hayes's ruling is that a man is legally dead when his brain no longer functions; thus the ruling brings the legal definition of death in line with the contemporary medical one.

Finally, it should be noted that almost everyone writing on this subject today insists that the doctors who declare a patient dead must not be connected with any transplant surgery which is to take place. This is a wise caution and good common sense. There should be no grounds for suspicion that a hasty declaration of death has been pronounced for any reason. A man should be declared dead only because he is dead, not because his organs are needed for transplantation.

At the same time, a man should be declared dead when he is dead and should not be made to respirate and circulate blood mechanically when he is a corpse. Needlessly prolonged sustenance of respiration and heartbeat can be a cause of expense and emotional pain to the family as well as an affront to the dignity of a man who has already died.

Selection of the Organ Recipient

The problem of the equitable distribution of sparse medical resources will always be with us in one form or another. Our sparsest resource today, relative to need, is organs for transplantation. For instance, more than fifty-thousand persons die each year from uremia due to kidney failure. About ten thousand of these could be saved either by the maintenance therapy of hemodialysis or by a kidney transplantation. But as a matter of fact, approximately seven thousand die because we lack sufficient resources to save them.[23]

The fundamental question here is that of determining our societal priorities. As Leibniz said, "All things are possible but all things are not compossible." We may be able to do anything, but we are not able to do everything. The fundamental question is whether or not the medical profession should be in the business of hemodialysis and kidney transplantation at all. Could the enormous amount of money and professional talent spent on these remedies better be used to prevent kidney disease? The answer to this larger question about the proper priorities for the allocation of our large but limited resources is far from clear. But it is the basic question, and it should be decided not by indecision but by rational social planning.

In any event, at the present time we have to face the hard practical question: When all cannot be saved, who should be chosen to live and who should be allowed to die? And specifically, what criteria should be used in deciding who should receive a needed transplant and who should not?

First of all, it is reasonable to screen out certain patients on strictly medical grounds. At the outset strictly medical criteria should be applied. No one should be considered a candidate for a transplant unless he is in critical need of one and there is reasonable hope that such an operation would bestow some significant benefit on him. A patient who is too ill to survive or benefit from the operation should be excluded as a candidate for a transplant. So should a patient who has some systemic disease which would soon destroy the newly implanted organ. It will also sometimes be necessary to make discriminating judgments among various patients according to the chance of success for each of them. Because of age or mental attitude, some will be less likely to benefit from transplant surgery than others.

Tissue matching is also an important consideration. Tissues are typed or classified according to their leukocyte antigens, somewhat in the same way as blood is typed according to sera and cell. There is good reason to believe that when a donor is unrelated, the selection of a recipient on the basis of tissue match can improve the prognosis.

Medical criteria like these should first be employed. But after they have been applied and some patients have been screened out on medical grounds, the problem of who should receive the organ frequently will not be resolved. There will still be more medically suitable candidates for transplants than there are organs available. Further criteria for selection are necessary, and two have been suggested. One is that patients should be chosen according to their social worth. The other is that they should be chosen by lot or on a first-come, first-served basis.

Selection of those to be saved on the basis of social worth or utility is not without precedent. In 1943 there was a shortage of penicillin among the United States armed forces in North Africa. It was needed for the treatment of victims of venereal disease and victims of battle wounds. The decision of the theatre medical commander was to give the penicillin to those wounded in brothels rather than to those wounded in battle. The reason for his decision was that those wounded in brothels could more quickly be restored to fighting capacity. The ability to make war was the most urgent need and best served the common good.

Triage in disaster medicine follows the same principle. Those most in need of help are quietly set aside, and attention is given first to those who can quickly be restored to functioning capability, since everyone's efforts are needed in the common purpose of survival.

In these cases the necessary goals can be easily identified, and social worth and usefulness can be realistically measured.

But life is rarely like that. In our pluralistic society we do not have one or several unanimously agreed upon goals, nor do we have a clear consensus on what sort of life or person is worth more to society than another.

In investigating what actually happens when committees select patients for medical treatment on the basis of social worth, David Sanders and Jesse Dukeminier found "a disturbing picture of the bourgeoisie sparing the bourgeoisie," and remarked that "the Pacific Northwest is no place for a Henry David Thoreau with bad kidneys."[24] One wonders how much chance an artist or composer would have before most committees in competition with a mother of five children.

When a society's goals are not simple and clearly focused, attempts to choose who should live and who should not on the basis of social worth or usefulness will seldom be successful, especially since cultural values are not the same as genuine social values, and since the estimate of the value of a man's life that has to be made will necessarily be filtered through the biases of those enlisted to make the choice.

The other option is random selection, either by lot or on a first-come, first-served basis. There is legal precedent for random selection of those to be saved when all cannot be saved. It is the rule in United States maritime law. In the *United States* v. *Holmes* it was ruled that in the desperate situation of an overloaded lifeboat, the decision on who should be saved and who abandoned must be made by lot. It was argued that a lottery is the only means of selection which avoids arbitrariness and shows respect for equal rights to life.

My first reaction to the plan of selecting patients for transplants by lot was that it was an abdication of the human responsibility for making a hard rational decision. At worst, I thought, it was a superstitious parody of the idea of leaving the decision "in the hands of God"; at best, it was decision by refusal to decide at a time when the best possible human decision was called for. When either of these is the mentality behind random selection, then of course it is unconscionable. But there is a deeper and wiser principle here.

Random selection of those to be saved when all cannot be saved cuts to the heart of the issue. It says that the human person is of transcendental value, that the value of a human life transcends one's usefulness or social worth. On this deeper level all lives should be respected equally and each one given an equal chance.

As a general policy, therefore, after some patients have been screened out on strictly medical grounds, selection of those who will receive a transplant should be made randomly, on a first-come, first-served basis or by lot. One cannot say that this rule is absolute and admits of no exceptions, but as a general policy it is the most equitable and fair. It is founded on the belief that the true value of a person's life cannot be calculated in utilitarian terms, that at its deepest level every human life has a meaning and value which go beyond its usefulness and social worth, and that, as a matter of fact, a man's social worth can seldom be rightly measured in a pluralistic society with unfocused values and goals.

CHAPTER 3

HUMAN EXPERIMENTATION

Medical research is essential to the development and expansion of medical knowledge, and sound medical research ultimately requires experimentation on human beings. Most of the standard medical and surgical procedures in use today were once highly experimental. Contemporary men are in debt to past experimental research, and future men will be in debt to the experiments of today.

Scientific medical knowledge, however, is not the only value nor is it the highest value, to which all other values are subordinate. The human person does not exist for the common good. He is an end in himself and cannot be thought of or used as only a means to some higher good or to the greater good of a larger society. This means that there are some moral limits to experimentation on man.

The totalitarian attitude toward man did not die with the deaths of the Nazi war criminals. Professional medical journals still carry accounts of human experimentation that show no concern for the welfare or dignity of the human subjects.[1] Dr. Henry K. Beecher has pointed out one of the problems: "Every young man knows that he will never be promoted to a tenure post, to a professorship in a major medical school, unless he has proved himself as an investigator. If the ready availability of money for conducting research is added to this fact, one can see how great the pressures are on ambitious young physicians."[2]

To say that there are a considerable number of abuses in human experimentation is not to indict the whole enterprise of medical research. On the whole it is morally excellent. The horrifying events disclosed at the Nuremberg trials have sensitized the conscience of the medical profession as well as that of the rest of the world to the dehumanizing results of a totalitarian view of man.

In June 1964 the World Medical Association adopted a set of guidelines for doctors involved in clinical research. It is known as the *Declaration of Helsinki*. It has been endorsed by the American Federation for Clinical Research, the American Society for Clinical Investigation, the Central Society for Clinical Research, the American College of Physicians, the American College of Surgeons, the Society for Pediatric Research, the American Academy of Pediatrics, and the American Medical Association. It is an excellent moral code and it deserves to be quoted in full.

Declaration of Helsinki

INTRODUCTION

It is the mission of the doctor to safeguard the health of the people. His knowledge and conscience are dedicated to the fulfillment of this mission.

The Declaration of Geneva of the World Medical Association binds the doctor with the words: "The health of my patient will be my first consideration" and the International Code of Medical Ethics which declares that "Any act or advice which could weaken physical or mental resistance of a human being may be used only in his interest."

Because it is essential that the results of laboratory experiments be applied to human beings to further scientific knowledge and to help suffering humanity, the World Medical Association has prepared the following recommendations as a guide to each doctor in clinical research. It must be stressed that the standards as drafted are only a guide to physicians all over the world. Doctors are not relieved from criminal, civil, and ethical responsibilities under the laws of their own countries.

In the field of clinical research a fundamental distinction must be recognized between clinical research in which the aim is essentially therapeutic for a patient, and the clinical research, the essential object of which is purely scientific and without therapeutic value to the person subjected to the research.

I. BASIC PRINCIPLES

1. Clinical research must conform to the moral and scientific principles that justify medical research and should be based on laboratory and animal experiments or other scientifically established facts.
2. Clinical research should be conducted only by scientifically qualified persons and under the supervision of a qualified medical man.
3. Clinical research cannot legitimately be carried out unless the importance of the objective is in proportion to the inherent risk to the subject.
4. Every clinical research project should be preceded by careful assessment of inherent risks in comparison to foreseeable benefits to the subject or to others.
5. Special caution should be exercised by the doctor in performing clinical research in which the personality of the subject is liable to be altered by drugs or experimental procedure.

II. CLINICAL RESEARCH COMBINED WITH PROFESSIONAL CARE

1. In the treatment of the sick person, the doctor must be free to use a new therapeutic measure, if in his judgment it offers hope of saving life, reestab-

lishing health, or alleviating suffering. If at all possible, consistent with patient psychology, the doctor should obtain the patient's freely given consent after the patient has been given a full explanation. In case of legal incapacity, consent should also be procured from the legal guardian; in case of physical incapacity, the permission of the legal guardian replaces that of the patient.

2. The doctor can combine clinical research with professional care, the objective being the acquisition of new medical knowledge, only to the extent that clinical research is justified by its therapeutic value for the patient.

III. NON-THERAPEUTIC CLINICAL RESEARCH

1. In the purely scientific application of clinical research carried out on a human being, it is the duty of the doctor to remain the protector of the life and health of that person on whom clinical research is being carried out.
2. The nature, the purpose, and the risk of clinical research must be explained to the subject by the doctor.
3 a. Clinical research on a human being cannot be undertaken without his free consent after he has been informed; if he is legally incompetent, the consent of the legal guardian should be procured.
   b. The subject of clinical research should be in such a mental, physical, and legal state as to be able to exercise fully his power of choice.
   c. Consent should, as a rule, be obtained in writing. However, the responsibility for clinical research always remains with the research worker; it never falls on the subject even after consent is obtained.

4. a. The investigator must respect the right of each individual to safeguard his personal integrity, especially if the subject is in a dependent relationship to the investigator.

   b. At any time during the course of clinical research the subject or his guardian should be free to withdraw permission for research to be continued.

   The investigator or the investigating team should discontinue the research if in his or their judgment, it may, if continued, be harmful to the individual.

Informed Consent

In a sense every medical procedure is experimental. Giving an antibiotic to see if it will lower a fever or performing a barium X-ray to determine the cause of internal bleeding are experiments, since their outcome is not absolutely certain. Also, every medical procedure entails some risk. There is risk in major or minor surgery. There is risk in the administration of anesthetics and drugs. There is even risk that a baby will be dropped on its head when being weighed.

Nonetheless, most of these procedures are so tested and established that we can be fairly certain of their results. They may be considered therapeutic rather than experimental procedures even though there is some possibility that they will not work or will be harmful. Truly experimental procedures, on the other hand, are those which have not been so thoroughly tested or established, so that their outcome is problematic.

Sometimes experimental measures are taken for the benefit of the patient. If established measures do not work or are not available, it is reasonable for the physician to use some other, less certain, measures to try to cure his patient. Even if the procedure is risky, it is reasonable to use it as long as the amount of risk is not disproportionate to the good that is hoped for.

There is little danger of abuse when the purpose of experimentation is to benefit the patient. A doctor whose interest is solely the welfare of his patient will not prescribe unestablished or dangerous treatments when orthodox and safe means are available. He will take no unnecessary chances and will assume only those risks that are warranted by the need of his patient.

The danger of abuse is in experimentation that is done not for the specific benefit of the patient but for the benefit of others, i.e., for the expansion of medical knowledge. Here a tension arises between two important goals—the advancement of medical science and the protection of the rights, dignity, and security of the individual.

Dr. Beecher describes the problem succinctly: "Every act of a doctor designed soundly to relieve or cure a given patient is experimentation of an easily justifiable kind. The patient's placement of himself in the doctor's hands is evidence of consent. The problem becomes a knotty one when the acts of the physician are directed not toward benefit of the patient present but toward patients in general. Such action requires the explicit consent of the *informed* patient."[3]

The tribunal of Nuremberg, Pope Pius XII, the Declaration of Helsinki, the Ethical Guidelines for Clinical Investigation of the AMA, and every other ethical code insist that no experimentation be undertaken without the informed consent of the subject. The investigator and the subject are joint partners in the experiment. As Paul Ramsey points out, "Just as Lincoln said . . . that 'no man is good enough to govern another without his consent,' so . . . no man is good enough to experiment upon another without his consent."[4]

However, it is one thing to affirm the necessity of getting informed consent; it is quite another thing to get it in practice. When is the subject fully informed? How can an experimenter adequately explain risks that he himself often does not know? How does he give an adequate explanation to the layman, the uneducated, the mentally incompetent, to children, or a fetus?

And when is consent truly free and voluntary? Even if no violence is exerted, cannot consent be subtly coerced and engineered? How free are such captive populations as prisoners, the poor in county hospitals, servicemen, or the students of an experimenting professor? How free are patients who are in a dependent relationship with the doctor?

Because of the practical problems involved in insuring valid consent in such cases, a number of doctors and ethicists argue that no experiments should be performed on children, mental incompetents, or captive populations. The only exception to this rule would be made for those experiments which carry no risk at all. If medical students are to be used, they should never be asked to be subjects by their own professors or by anyone having power over them. The rationale behind this strict posture is that it is better to set limits to medical experimentation than to risk experimenting on anyone without his informed and free consent.

Hans Jonas has proposed a "rule of descending order." He writes: "The poorer in knowledge, motivation, and freedom of decision (and that, alas, means the more readily available in terms of numbers and possible manipulation), the more sparingly and indeed reluctantly should the reservoir be used, and the more compelling must therefore become the countervailing justification."[5] At the least, extreme caution must always be used, and if a mistake is to be made, it should be made in favor of the human subject rather than of medical science and the common good.

The Responsible Investigator

As a practical matter it is clear that no detailed code or set of rules can be formulated which will substitute for the personal judgment of the responsible investigator. Nothing is more important in this area than the moral sensitivity and integrity of the investigator.

As the British Medical Research Council has pointed out, it is not enough merely to obtain the consent of the subject. Rather, "owing to the special relationship of trust that exists between a patient and his doctor, most patients will consent to any proposal that is made. Further, the considerations involved in a novel procedure are nearly always so technical as to prevent their being adequately understood by one who is not himself an expert. It must, therefore, be frankly recognized that, for practical purposes, an inescapable moral responsibility rests with the doctor concerned for determining what investigations are, or are not, proposed to a particular patient or volunteer."[6] Similarly, after stressing the importance of obtaining valid consent, Dr. Beecher says that there is a second and more dependable requirement, namely "the presence of an informed, intelligent, skillful, compassionate, responsible investigator."[7]

The responsible investigator will always follow the golden rule. He will never exploit the dependent and trusting relationship, the weakness, or the ignorance of his patients. He will not choose martyrs for science and will be acutely aware that good results do not justify an unethical experiment. As Dr. Beecher observes, "An experiment does not become ethical *post hoc;* it is ethical at its inception, or it is not."[8]

Part Two

Human Sexuality

CHAPTER 4

CONTRACEPTION AND STERILIZATION

In his famous encyclical of 1968, *Humanae Vitae,* Pope Paul VI reaffirmed the historic Catholic teaching that each and every act of sexual intercourse must remain open to the transmission of life. Birth control by means of the "rhythm method," i.e., abstinence from sexual intercourse during the fertile period, is morally permissible. But every other form of contraception and sterilization is always forbidden.

Pope Paul said: "These acts, by which husband and wife are united in chaste intimacy, and by means of which human life is transmitted, are, as the council recalled, 'noble and worthy,' and they do not cease to be lawful if, for causes independent of the will of husband and wife, they are foreseen to be infecund, since they always remain ordained toward expressing and consolidating their union. In fact, as experience bears witness, not every conjugal act is followed by a new life. God has wisely disposed natural laws and rhythms of fecundity which, of themselves, cause a separation in the succession of births. Nonetheless the church, calling men back to the observance of the norms of the natural law, as interpreted by their constant doctrine, teaches that each and every marriage act must remain open to the transmission of life."[1]

Therefore the pope condemns as absolutely illicit "direct sterilization, whether perpetual or temporary, whether of the man or of the woman" and "every action which, either in anticipation of the conjugal act, or in its accomplishment, or in the development of its natural consequences, proposes, whether as an end or as a means, to render procreation impossible."[2]

For a long time Catholic moral theologians have tried earnestly to defend these conclusions, but in recent years they have found them increasingly difficult to sustain. Contemporary moral analysis is still divided. But today, I think it is fair to say, a clear and decisive majority of Catholic moralists no longer support the traditional doctrine.

The new consensus does not deny that there is an essential connection between the procreative and love-union aspects of sexual intercourse. It affirms that these two aspects must be maintained in principle. Sexual intercourse is not only lovemaking; it is also life-giving. God's creative love is mirrored in human procreative loving. As God's love is creative—he created nothing apart from his love—so we create new beings like ourselves in the midst of our love for one another. Sexual love is a special kind of love, the kind that is creative of new human life. To separate in principle the lovemaking and life-giving aspects of sexual intercourse is to refuse the image of God's creative love in human procreative loving.

What this means is that sexual intercourse has an essential relationship to parenthood. But it does not mean that each individual act must be open to the transmission of life. The link between sex and parenthood is to be maintained. But it is not to be maintained blindly, with the decision of whether or not to procreate new life left entirely in the hands of chance or divine providence. Human parents must make responsible rational decisions about the number and spacing of their children. There may have been a time in human history when quantitative reproduction of the species was the paramount value, but that is no longer the case. Today quantitative reproduction is seen as a disvalue in our overpopulated world. The quality of life is now the most important consideration.

In the early sixties Catholic moralists began to question the Church's condemnation of oral contraceptives. Their analysis of the morality of the use of the pill forced them to enlarge their inquiry to include every form or method of contraception. The majority conclusion at the end of the sixties was that the method used for contraception was morally irrelevant. In ethical terms it does not matter what method or technique is used for birth control. All that matters is that the link between human sexual love and parenthood not be broken in principle and that the practical decision about the number and spacing of children be made unselfishly and with responsible concern for the quality of engendered human life.

Linked with this new ethical analysis of contraception, and in some measure a result of it, was a new theology of dissent which was developed by Catholic ecclesiologists. Post-Vatican I ecclesiology held that no one might licitly disagree with an authoritative decision of the ordinary papal magisterium except an expert in the field who had uncovered some new evidence in his research—and even the expert was only to suspend his judgment while he secretly brought the new evidence to the attention of the Holy See. Contemporary ecclesiology affirms the right of any person to dissent from noninfallible decisions of the Church when he has sufficient reason for doing so.

There can be many good reasons why people should practice birth control. Respect for human life means respect for the quality of human life and not just its quantitative reproduction. Responsible parenthood means more than generous procreation. It also means the feeding, clothing, housing, and education of children. In our society at least a high-school education is necessary if a person is to live with any dignity, and it is quite reasonable for parents to want to provide a college education for their sons and daughters. To fulfill the duties consequent upon procreation, parents must spend a large amount of money.

The physical health of the mother is often an important consideration in deciding responsibly for or against another pregnancy. The nervous state and mental health of the contemporary housewife have become increasingly important. Add the strains of modern life to the strain of raising children today and you will understand why there are women on every block who are nervous wrecks and many who have already been hospitalized for nervous breakdowns.

There is also the larger problem of overpopulation. Many competent demographers and economists predict that within a few centuries the human race will be facing disaster. This prediction is challenged by other experts who think that the food problem can be solved by the use of fertilizers, by tripling the present area of arable land, by making food through photosynthesis of algae, and, most importantly, by solving the real problem, which is not production but distribution of food. But even if the more optimistic experts are correct—and they may not be—even if technological man can prevent a demographic disaster for a number of centuries, the fact remains that large numbers of people in many areas of the world are already suffering from starvation and overcrowding and that without birth control *now*, human lives will continue to be dehumanized.

Methods of Controlling Birth

A simple and common method of avoiding pregnancy without any mechanical devices or chemicals is the technique of Onan, *coitus interruptus* or withdrawal. Before ejaculation the man withdraws his penis from the vagina.

There are a number of problems with this method: intercourse before orgasm cannot be relaxed; it is frustrating for the man to withdraw at the very moment when his natural impulse is to drive his penis deeply into the vagina; the woman often does not reach orgasm; and, since timing is so important the method is not always effective. The first few drops of ejaculate contain most of the spermatozoa; the secretion of the Cowper's glands sometimes contains sperm; and because some sperm is left in the urethra after ejaculation, reunion then would be dangerous. Withdrawal is considered to be between 92 percent and 60 percent effective in preventing conception, depending on the carefulness and timing of the man.

Another method is condomistic intercourse. A condom or "rubber" is a cone-shaped bag made of rubber or sheep's intestine. It is about 1½ inches in diameter and about 7½ inches long. If it does not have a small pocket at the end to catch and hold the semen, the user should leave about a half-inch loose at the end to prevent breakage. The user should also check it for holes before use either by blowing in it or, preferably, by filling it with water. About seven hundred and fifty million condoms are produced each year in the United States. They are used more frequently in nonmarital intercourse and are very effective in the prevention of venereal disease. The condom does not dull pleasure appreciably unless it is coated with too much lubrication. There is always some danger of its breaking in use or slipping off, or of semen trickling out after the penis has become soft. In general, the condom is considered to be about 89 percent effective in preventing conception.

There are two main types of contraceptive pessaries, the cervical cap and the diaphragm. The cervical cap is a metal, rubber, or plastic cap that fits over the cervix and blocks the entrance of sperm into the uterus. It must be fitted by a physician and is kept in place partly by suction. It is generally used together with spermicidal creams or jellies. Since rubber caps can be worn for only twenty-four hours, most cervical caps are made of plastic; these can remain in place throughout the time between menstrual periods. They are used more commonly in Europe than in the United States. They are difficult for the woman to insert and remove, and when they are left in place, they sometimes have a tendency to migrate. They are about 96 percent to 90 percent effective.

The diaphragm is one of the most popular contraceptive devices in use today. Many women are returning to its use because of the scare about the pill or because of their own bad experience with the pill. The diaphragm is a piece of rubber stretched over a collapsible metal ring. It is inserted in the vagina so as to occlude the mouth of the uterus. It should be used together with spermicidal creams or jellies. It must be fitted the first time by a physician; after that the woman can learn to insert and remove it herself. It is inserted immediately or several hours before intercourse and may not be removed until about six hours afterward. It may be left in place for as long as twenty-four hours. When used with spermicidal chemicals it is about 96 percent to 90 percent effective.

Another very effective instrument is the intrauterine contraceptive device (IUCD). This is a small loop, spiral, bow, or ring made out of plastic (or sometimes metal). It is inserted into the uterus and left there. A thin string attached to it hangs down through the vagina so that the woman can occasionally check to see if it is still in place. How, precisely, it prevents pregnancy is not entirely clear. Some few medical authroities think that it causes peristalsis of the Fallopian tubes, so that the released ovum travels through the tubes and uterus too quickly to be fertilized. What appears to be the case is that it interferes with nidation. In some way it renders the complex process of implantation impossible; hence its effect is contraimplantation rather than contraception. Although it sometimes causes bleeding and pain and sometimes is rejected by the uterus, it is so simple, cheap, and effective that Dr. Alan Guttmacher predicts that it will be the most important contraceptive for the immediate, foreseeable future. It is rated between 99 percent and 97 percent effective.

Spermicidal chemicals are also used. They generally come in the form of creams, jellies, and foams. Vaginal suppositories that melt after about fifteen minutes or vaginal tablets that dissolve in moisture may also be used. These chemicals must be inserted into the vagina from five to fifteen minutes before ejaculation occurs. They are considered to be between 95 percent and 73 percent effective. The new foams in aerosol spray cans can easily be spread all around the vagina and are between 97 percent and 90 percent effective.

Vaginal douches are relatively ineffectual and are rated only about 64 percent effective. The vagina is flushed out after intercourse with plain water or with a solution such as vinegar, soapsuds, or alum. Other devices sometimes used—such as sponges, tampons, or balls of cotton treated with spermicides—are also relatively ineffective. Their rating is about 73 percent to 68 percent.

The most effective means of contraception is sterilization. The male can be sterilized by a simple surgical operation performed under local anesthesia in the physician's office. The operation is called a vasectomy. An incision is made on both sides of the scrotum above the testicles, an inch of the vas deferens is excised, and the two ends are tied. Since no more sperm can be carried to the seminal vesicles and those already present will die after a short time, fertility will come to an end after several days. After the operation the patient is not incapacitated, but should avoid strenuous work or exerçise for about two days. If the operation is done skillfully, spontaneous recanalization rarely takes place.

The man normally suffers no impotency or decrease of sexual desire. Two hundred thousand vasectomies are performed each year in the United States, and the procedure should become more widespread as some of the myths that surround it are laid to rest. If for some reason a man regrets his decision, it is sometimes possible to repair the vasectomy. Today there is about a 50 percent chance of success in an attempt to restore fertility through surgical recanalization of the tubes.

Castration, the surgical removal of the testicles, is a more drastic method of sterilization. It often results in changes in secondary sex characteristics, which, however, can be controlled by hormone therapy. It does not necessarily result in impotence if it is performed on an adult. But if one's only purpose is sterilization, a vasectomy is the preferred technique.

Surgical sterilization of the female is a more complicated procedure. There are a number of techniques currently in use. An oophorectomy is the surgical excision of both ovaries. After the ovaries have been removed, no more ova will be produced, and hormone therapy is sometimes needed to prevent changes in secondary sex characteristics. A salpingectomy is a surgical operation in which the Fallopian tubes are cut, tied, and resectioned. It is easily done and is often recommended by doctors during a Caesarean section. The operation is considered about 99 percent effective or better in preventing pregnancy. It is possible to attempt to rejoin the tubes so as to restore fertility, but the operation is risky and the chance of success is small. Work is presently in progress on a simpler technique in which metal or plastic clamps are attached to the tubes by way of a small incision in the vagina.

A technique which is used frequently in Japan and which probably will receive more attention in the United States is intrauterine coagulation of the uterine tube outlet. The openings of the tubes into the uterus are electrically cauterized, and the resulting scar tissue permanently blocks the tubular orifices.

A hysterectomy, i.e., the surgical removal of the uterus, is generally performed through the vagina. It is seldom performed solely for the purpose of sterilization.

Birth control pills are probably best classified as sterilizing drugs, since sterilization is their primary effect, although they also seem to work as contraceptives and abortifacients. The pills are a combination of synthetic hormones (progesterone and estrogen) which has three effects: (1) it inhibits the production of pituitary gonadotropin and so inhibits the growth and development of the ovarian follicles (sterilization); (2) it affects the mucous lining of the uterus so as to make implantation more difficult and early spontaneous abortion more likely if conception does take place (abortion); and (3) it causes the mucous plug of the cervix to thicken so as to keep sperm from entering the uterus (contraception).

A woman starts taking the pills on the fifth day after the first day of menstruation. She takes one each day, preferably at the same hour, for twenty days. Menstruation will usually occur two to five days after the last pill is taken. Five days after the menstruation begins, she starts the cycle of pills again, and so on until she no longer wishes to be infertile. If menstruation does not occur after she has taken the twenty pills, she simply begins taking them again after seven days. When taken according to instructions, oral contraceptives are practically 100 percent effective in preventing pregnancy.

The pill, of course, is often prescribed for therapeutic purposes other than the suppression of fertility—for instance, as a remedy for premenstrual tension, excessive bleeding, an irregular menstrual cycle, and certain skin disorders.

Another method of controlling birth is to abstain from sexual intercourse during the female's fertile days of the month. This is known as the safe period or rhythm method. A woman generally ovulates about once a month. The ovum lives for about twenty-four hours after ovulation, and the sperm can live in the uterus for about forty-eight hours. Therefore conception is possible only during three days of the month.

Ovulation is generally believed to take place fourteen to sixteen days before menstruation. Therefore to determine the time of ovulation, a woman must count back from the first day of her next anticipated menstruation. By counting back sixteen days she arrives at the earliest time of ovulation, and by counting back fourteen days she arrives at the latest time of ovulation. If she has a twenty-eight-day menstrual cycle, she will ovulate between the thirteenth and fifteenth day after the first day of her period. Allowing for the life span of the ovum and the sperm, she should abstain from coitus from the eleventh to the seventeenth days after the first day of her last menstruation.

If a woman has an irregular menstrual cycle, she should keep written records of the time of menstruation for one year in order to determine the earliest and the latest time of menstruation. For instance, if her cycle varies between twenty-four and twenty-eight days, by counting back sixteen from the earliest time of the next menstruation and fourteen from the latest time of the next menstruation, she can determine the earliest time of ovulation (eight days after the first day of the last period) and the latest time of ovulation (fifteen days after the first day of the last period). Adding time for the viability of the sperm and egg, she can determine that conception will be possible between the sixth and seventeenth days after the beginning of her menstrual period.

Aside from the emotional or psychological difficulties that sometimes result from abstinence during the fertile or unsafe period, there are also some technical problems with this method. Certain emotions, such as fear or joy, can postpone or hasten ovulation. After childbirth the first few months are frequently too irregular for any safe period to be calculated, and during menopause the menstrual cycle is generally too irregular to permit reliable calculations of fertile periods. About 15 percent of all women have cycles too irregular for the use of this method.

Another method of determining the time of ovulation is by measurement of basal temperature, or lowest normal body temperature of the day. At the time of ovulation or one or two days after there is a dip in temperature and then a sharp rise of $^{1}/_{2}$ to $^{7}/_{10}$ of a degree; the temperature remains at this higher level until one or two days before the beginning of the next period. Since the ovum lives only for one or two days, after this rise in temperature no conception is possible for the rest of that cycle. A woman should keep a record of her temperature in the morning for about six months in order to determine any peculiarities. One of the problems with this method is that other factors, such as a cold, can also cause a rise in temperature and so confuse the pattern. Further, it is possible for more than one ovum to mature during a cycle.

Because of the polemics that have surrounded the question of rhythm or periodic continence as the "Catholic" method of birth control, it is difficult to ascertain how effective it really is. Some authorities rate it as 86 percent effective; others make higher claims. Contemporary research no doubt will increase its effectiveness. Recently Prof. Jacques Ferin of the Belgian University of Louvain announced that thanks to technological progress, doctors are very close to being able to predict with certainty the day on which a woman could conceive during her menstrual cycle.[3] Dr. Mary S. Calderone has said: "Stop apologizing for the rhythm method. We have a tendency to . . . list all of the medical methods, and then say, with a shrug, 'and the rhythm method.' Well, we should know the facts about it: it is very effective. . . . You're going to have failures with practically any method, but you are certainly going to have failures with the rhythm method, not because it is not effective, but because the restrictions it places on people make it rate low in acceptability."[4]

For the record we might note another method known as Carezza, or as it is called in most of the moral literature, *amplexus reservatus.* This is the prolongation of coitus, even for hours, without male ejaculation. It does not seem to have gained much popularity.

The Theological Argument

The argument made against contraception by Pope Paul VI in *Humanae Vitae* is the same as that made in the recent past by theologians like Josef Fuchs. Fuchs, of course, changed his opinion during the study and discussions of the papal birth control commission, and he expressed his revised opinion in the majority report.

The principal ethical argument against contraception is based on an analysis of the act of sexual intercourse as an expression of a love relationship which is totally self-giving and procreative in character. Fuchs developed the argument in this way: "The Creator so arranged the sexual act that it is simultaneously both per se generative and per se expressive of intimate oblative love. He has so arranged it that procreation would take place from an act intimately expressive of conjugal love and that this act expressive of conjugal love would tend toward procreation. Therefore an act which *of itself* does not appear to be apt for procreation is by this very fact shown to be one which does not conform to the intentions of the Creator. The same thing should be said about an act which *of itself* is not apt for the expression of oblative love. Indeed, an act which is not apt for procreation is by this very fact shown to be one which is *of itself* not apt for the expression of conjugal love; for the sexual act is one."[5]

This is the same argument that found its way into *Humanae Vitae,* in which Pope Paul wrote: "That teaching often set forth by the magisterium is founded upon the inseparable connection, established by God and unable to be broken by man on his own initiative, between the unitive and procreative meanings, both of which are present in the conjugal act. For by this intimate structure, the conjugal act, while most closely uniting husband and wife, also capacitates them for the generation of new life, according to laws inscribed in the very being of man and woman. By safeguarding both of these essential aspects, the unitive and the procreative, the use of marriage preserves in its fullness the sense of true mutual love and its ordination to man's exalted calling to parenthood."[6]

Both the strength and the weakness of this argument are pointed up in the approach of Paul Ramsey. Ramsey affirms that sexual intercourse is at the same time an act of love and a procreative act. By this he does not mean that it always in fact nourishes love and engenders a child, but that it tends of its own nature toward strengthening of love (the unitive good) and engendering of children (the procreative good). This affirmation is not based on natural law in the sense of the mere fact and function of biological life, but on the Christian story of creation which appears not in the book of Genesis but in the Prologue to the Gospel of John and in Ephesians 5. Here we see that God created the entire world of his creatures out of love: God's love was creative and he created nothing apart from his love. Human love is made in the image of God's love. Human love reflects God's love because it is procreative. We procreate new beings like ourselves in the midst of our love for one another. In this there is a trace of the original mystery by which God created the world because of his love. Therefore, God's love is normative for Christian love. Hence a couple may not "procreate from beyond their marriage, or exercise love's one-flesh unity outside of it."[7]

Notice Ramsey's conclusion. He argues that man may not radically put asunder what God has joined together. But God made human love procreative. Therefore, Ramsey concludes not that contraception is illicit (that is what the pope concludes), but that artificial insemination and fornication are illicit, since by artificial insemination one procreates beyond the sphere of mutual love, and by fornication one loves beyond the sphere of responsible procreation. But by contraception the spheres of love and procreation are not separated, even though the act as unitive and procreative is divided.

The Catholic thesis, however, wants to conclude more from the premises. It wants to conclude that each act is unitive and procreative by God's design. Speaking of the separability of these two aspects of coitus as it has been defended by non-Catholics, Fuchs has argued: "They do not sufficiently grasp that the Creator *united* this double aspect. The sexual faculty has but *one* natural actuation in which the generative and oblative aspects specify each other." Others have contended that contraceptive interference cannot be viewed as a merely biological intervention. Rather, they argued, contraception does not permit the act to be procreative and *therefore* it does not permit the act to be expressive of personal love, either because it expresses some restriction in self-donation or because the permanent sign of this love, the child, is excluded. In other words, the marital act is essentially an act of procreative love. This is the act as given to us by God. If the married couple are to use it properly, they must allow the act to retain both of these essential characteristics.

In the past few years many theologians have found this analysis difficult to sustain. It is not easy to see why it is not sufficient to conclude, as Ramsey does, that the unitive and procreative goods may not be separated in principle but that separation is possible in an individual act. There are many acts of coitus that are in fact sterile and yet are expressive of personal love.

The central affirmation of *Humanae Vitae* is that because each marriage act must remain open to the transmission of life, every act of contraceptive intercourse is morally evil. It is fair to say that on the level of ethical analysis this affirmation remains unproven.

Papal teaching on this matter is not infallible doctrine. It is authentic noninfallible doctrine. It demands serious consideration and respect. But it does not exclude the possibility of error or rule out legitimate dissent.

Honesty in one's effort to come to a conscientious conclusion about contraception requires that one place under careful scrutiny one's own attitude toward ecclesiastical and magisterial authority. It is certainly bad theological methodology to go from the conclusion that the immorality of contraception is not infallibly taught to the presumption that it is therefore erroneous. One does not start with this presumption about authentic noninfallible teaching, but rather with the opposite.

Nonetheless, it is not easy to understand how the Holy Father could get the necessary certitude and clarity for the argument from reason. It is true that we must be wary, especially in moral matters, of the kind of rationalism that expects too much certitude from human reason, but neither can we assume that the pope receives his knowledge in some magical way.

A model of respectful dissent has been given by Richard

McCormick. In his "Notes on Moral Theology" he concludes: "In the light of these reflections it is the opinion of the compositor of these Notes that the intrinsic immorality of every contraceptive act remains a teaching subject to solid and positive doubt. This is not to say that this teaching of *Humanae Vitae* is certainly erroneous. It is only to say that there are very strong objections that can be urged against it and very little evidence that will sustain it. One draws this conclusion reluctantly and with no small measure of personal anguish. With proper allowance made for one's own shortcomings, pride, and resistance, what more can a theologian say? He can say, of course, that the teaching is clear and certain simply because the papal magisterium had said so. But ultimately such an assertion must rest on the supposition that the clarity and certainty of a conclusion of natural-law morality are independent of objective evidence."[8]

Sterilization

A great many priests and lay people no longer have any problems of conscience about artificial birth control. They have decided that papal teaching on contraception is either erroneous or at least solidly doubtful, and they are supported in their judgment by the common dissent of contemporary Catholic theologians. But frequently they do not have the same security or clarity of conscience on the question of sterilization.

Perhaps the reason for their hesitation here is that this specific question has not undergone the same kind of public debate and widespread airing in the media. Or perhaps the reason is that many priests are not so clear themselves on this issue. In seminary textbooks sterilization is not treated together with contraception. It is treated as a separate question in a separate section of the manuals. Contraception is treated under the sixth commandment as a sexual sin, whereas sterilization is treated under the fifth commandment as a sin of bodily mutilation.

The evil of sterilization, according to this argument, is that it is an unlawful mutilation of our bodies, since it involves the suppression of the function of a very important bodily faculty, the faculty by which we procreate new life. In all cases other than sterilization, mutilation is permitted if it is in accord with the principle of totality. That is to say, mutilation is permissible if done for the good of the whole body. For instance, an amputation is moral only if it is done for the total health of the individual. Since an arm or a leg is given by God for the good of the whole body, it may be sacrificed only for the good of the whole body.

The same reasoning, however, could not be applied to sterilization, the moralists argued, because unlike all other faculties and members of the human body, the sexual faculty is not given to us by God merely for the good of the whole body or individual person. The sexual faculty is given for the good of the species and so is not subordinated to the total good of any individual. The sexual faculty has a wider finality: it is ordered to the good of the human race.

When this traditional argument against sterilization was pressed, however, the real reason for opposition to the act was disclosed. The question was raised: If the sexual faculty is for the good of the species, may it be surgically excised or may its function be suppressed when necessary for the good of the species, for instance, in a population crisis? The response was negative. The reasoning: The sexual faculty is not for the good of the species in the sense that it is in any way subordinated to the common good or the good of society; rather, it is directly subordinated to God himself, the author of life.

Thus it became clear that the real objection to sterilization was the same as the objection to contraception in general. It interferes with the procreative purpose of sexual intercourse. Its fundamental evil is not that it is mutilation —if it were, it could be justified by the principle of totality. Its fundamental evil is that it is contraceptive mutilation. Hence, even if it is necessary for the total good or health of the individual, it is still intrinsically evil and therefore may not be willed, intended, or directly performed for any reason.

According to these principles only indirect sterilization is allowable. It would be morally permissible, for instance, to remove a cancerous uterus, even though sterilization would be a necessary but unintended consequence. But it is always forbidden to perform any surgical operation for the purpose of sterilization for any reason, even to protect the life or health of an individual or to safeguard any other important value. A good end never justifies an evil means. This is the theology contained in *Humanae Vitae,* in previous papal statements, and even in the American bishops' recent *Ethical and Religious Directives for Catholic Health Facilities.*

Contemporary moral analysis has found this thinking too narrow.[9] Sterilization that represents a rejection in principle of the relationship between human sexuality and parenthood is judged immoral. So is any form of contraception which would do the same thing. But sterilization done to protect some important value, for instance, one's health, marriage, or the quality of human life, is morally evaluated in the same way as contraception in general.

This means that in contemporary ethical thinking there is no essential moral difference between sterilization and other methods of birth control. Sterilization is contraceptive mutilation. Insofar as it is mutilation, it is governed by the principle of totality. Insofar as it is contraceptive, it is governed by the same principles as contraception. So long as it does not negate in principle the connection between sex and parenthood, it is permissible for a proportionate reason.

There are, however, some very important practical differences between sterilization and other contraceptive practices. One is the relative permanence of sterilization. In our swiftly changing world permanent decisions are risky. A young couple ought to be rather cautious when thinking about sterilization. Because of the current publicity vasectomies are fashionable now. But being fashionable now could prove later to be a grave and often irreparable mistake for a young married couple.

Many couples do not realize that there are other means of contraception which are generally as effective as sterilization and do not entail any irreversible decision. For instance, the use of a diaphragm, together with spermicidal foam sprayed over the vagina from an aerosol can, is about 96 percent effective. Also, the birth-control pill, properly used, is just as effective a means of preventing conception as a vasectomy.

An older couple, however, might reasonably make a different decision. Should they choose to terminate altogether and finally their reproductive capacity, their decision could more easily be considered prudent. This aspect of the issue should be carefully weighed in any individual decision.

There are two other practical considerations that might be mentioned. One is that because of its permanence a vasectomy or tubal ligation undergone before a marriage with the purpose of excluding all children would attack the *bonum prolis* in such a way as to affect the canonical validity of the marriage. The other practical consideration is the reported psychological effect that a vasectomy may have on a man. It is not easy to get accurate information about this, but it seems that at least in some cases a vasectomized man experiences a loss of his sense of male identity or masculinity. As far as I can tell this is not a usual result, but since it might occur, it should be at least a minor consideration in an individual's effort to come to a practical decision.

Voluntary sterilization, of course, is an issue quite separate from involuntary sterilization. A more difficult question arises concerning the mentally retarded.

A young girl in a mental institution may be so mentally deficient as to be completely unable to understand or cope with a pregnancy. Yet unless she is kept in isolation and under constant surveillance, there is a great likelihood that she will become pregnant.

Sterilization in this case could be justified by the principle of totality. It would be for the total good of the person that her reproductive capacity be ended. Since she could not give informed consent to sterilization, her parents or guardians would have to give it for her.

Some important cautions are needed here. Some retarded children are not so mentally deficient that they could not be loving parents capable of providing for and educating their children. Their life style might never attain the standards of middle-class suburbia. But that does not mean that the state or anyone else may deprive them of their right and ability to have children of their own.

No one should be sterilized involuntarily for the good of society, the taxpayers, or the hospital staff. An individual should be sterilized only if it is in his own interest and for his own good. Someone else will have to make this judgment for a child, and he or she will have to be extremely cautious in order to insure that it is being made honestly.

CHAPTER 5

TRANSSEXUALISM AND HOMOSEXUALITY

Transsexualism

According to one estimate there are about ten thousand transsexuals in the United States.[1] These are persons who have the anatomy of one sex and a psychological identification with the other. The cause of transsexualism is not altogether clear. Dr. Robert J. Stoller, a psychiatrist at the University of California, suggests that one's sexual identity is not set at birth but is conditioned in the first year or so by the surrounding environment. It is also possible that it may be influenced by a subtle imbalance in the hormone system. Whatever the cause or causes, the result is an inability to identify as a member of one's anatomical sex. The transsexual is physically male but feels and wants to be female, or vice versa.

At least by the time he begins school, the transsexual usually is trying to conform to the dress and behavior of his anatomical sex. Frequently he fails and is severely humiliated. He begins to live in a world of frustration and unreality. It is said that three out of ten transsexuals become so distraught that they commit suicide, while many others mutilate their sex organs.[2] Some, on the other hand, seek a transsexual operation. If the mind cannot be changed to fit the body, the body will be changed to fit the mind.

Transsexual operations have been performed in Europe since 1930. The most widely publicized case occurred in 1952, when George Jorgensen was changed to Christine. In 1966 Johns Hopkins Medical School opened its Gender Identity Clinic, and since then other centers have been opened in the United States to perform transsexual surgery.

At most centers applicants for surgery are carefully screened, and only those who show no signs of a psychosis are accepted. To change secondary sex characteristics hormonal therapy is prescribed for about a year. Administrations of estrogen and progesterone usually diminish hair and help to develop breasts and rounded hips, while androgens deepen the voice and stimulate the growth of a beard. During this period of hormonal treatment the candidate for transsexual surgery adopts the dress, life-style, and behavior patterns of the opposite sex. If the experience of living as a member of the opposite sex proves to be a happy one, surgery is finally performed.

Surgical transformation of males into females is a three- to four-hour operation costing from three thousand to five thousand dollars. The penis and testicles are amputated, and an artificial vagina is created, usually from the sensitive skin of the penis or the scrotum or from skin from the thigh or hip. The surgical transformation of females into males is rarer, more difficult, and two to three times as expensive. A hysterectomy is performed and the breasts are removed. Sometimes a miniature penis is made from the clitoris; sometimes a larger but practically insensitive penis is created from silicone forms and skin grafts from the abdomen.

Catholic moralists have in the past been unanimous in condemning transsexual surgery.[3] In the case of hermaphrodites they allowed a person to undergo surgery in order to become either one sex or the other. The only restriction they placed on hermaphrodites was that if one sex predominated over the other, the dominant sex had to be chosen. But a transsexual was never allowed to undergo surgery to change his anatomical sex.

Some authors argued that most transsexuals are in reality deeply disturbed homosexuals who are trying to resolve their inner conflicts by surgery. Others argued that if we allowed transsexuals to change their bodies to fit their minds, then "if a person were hopelessly convinced that he was a monkey or a dog, should we not dedicate our surgical skills toward making him look like a monkey or a dog to relieve his psychological frustration?"[4]

Such arguments are obviously unfair. There is little evidence to support the view that transsexuals are in reality homosexuals, and no legitimate comparison can be made between transsexuals and psychotic individuals who think they are dogs. The true transsexual is simply an otherwise normal person who cannot identify with his anatomical sex because of prenatal hormonal influence or early environmental conditioning.

Behind the older moralists' absolute prohibition against transsexual surgery was the same premise that led them to absolutely forbid direct sterilization. Transsexual surgery, after all, is a sterilizing operation, and direct sterilization was always considered by these authors as intrinsically evil. It could never be justified by the principle of totality because the sexual faculty has a wider finality than the good of the individual: it is also for the good of the species.

As we have seen, contemporary moral analysis questions this reasoning.[5] Many Catholic theologians today argue that sterilization is justified by the principle of totality: direct sterilization is permissible when it is done for the welfare of the whole person.

There has been little contemporary ethical discussion of transsexual surgery, but it seems to me that it is subject to the same kind of analysis as sterilization. In itself transsexual surgery is a disvalue. So is every form of surgery or physical mutilation. But in certain circumstances it is permissible in order to achieve a greater good.

This means that if transsexual surgery is medically indicated, it is morally licit. If in certain circumstances it is necessary for the total well-being of an individual, it is morally permissible according to the principle of totality.

In trying to evaluate what constitutes the total well-being of an individual, one must be extremely cautious. For one thing, it is quite unlikely that anyone who has undergone transsexual surgery can ever be canonically married in the Catholic Church. Moreover, transsexual surgery is no trivial thing; it is a rather extreme, drastic, and irrevocable measure which should be undertaken only as a last resort.

Homosexuality

A good number of psychiatrists and psychologists no longer classify homosexuality as a pathological condition. They argue that it warrants treatment only when it is personally disturbing to the individual. Others still maintain that it is in itself an abnormality. There is no way for me to resolve this debate in the medical profession or to know for certain which view is true. Nonetheless, some homosexuals do experience inner conflict because of their condition and come to doctors for help, and therefore an ethical analysis of homosexuality may be useful.

The meaning that one attaches to human sexuality will depend to a large extent on one's view of man. A dualistic anthropology which thinks of man as a spiritual person who has a material body will be inclined to undervalue man's sexuality. As we use our bodies, so we use our sexuality. Sex can be used for various purposes—for the expression of love and affection, for procreation, or for fun and pleasure.

But one who believes that man is his body, that he is the body of his soul as well as the soul of his body, will be more inclined to see the use of sex as expressive of his person. Sex is the way that he, who is his body, does the two most important things in life—loving and creating other beings like himself.

Human sexuality is both lovemaking and life-giving. That is its full human and Christian meaning, and anything less diminishes it. On the objective level homosexuality is something less. Homosexual acts are not life-giving acts of love. They separate in principle the love-union and procreative aspects of human sexuality. That is why Christians have always condemned them.

It is possible for two persons of the same sex to truly love one another in the deepest sense of the word. A genuine love relationship is more unusual between male homosexuals than between lesbians. It is at least statistically true that most male homosexual relationships are casual affairs, and it is rare that any kind of permanent bond rooted in interpersonal love is established. Female homosexuals, on the other hand, more frequently establish a permanent relationship based on genuine mutual love.

Nonetheless, a truly permanent loving relationship is not enough to fulfill the meaning of sexual communion. Good as love is, sexual union means more. Homosexuals may use sex to express love, but sex is more than an act of love. It is an act of creative love, an act by which we love and create new beings like ourselves.

An older theology exaggerated the importance of procreation and undervalued the importance of love. Procreation was seen as the primary end of sex, and any other values stood in a subordinate position. What we have to watch out for today is an overcorrection of this view, one which would dismiss procreation as if it were wholly irrelevant to the meaning of human sexuality.

Contemporary theological analysis no longer says that procreation is the principal purpose of sex, nor does it say that each and every act must be procreative or open to the transmission of life. It does not analyze our sexuality as a purely biological function. It sees it as a human function and says that as a human function it still has an essential relation to procreation.

Human sexuality is not just for loving. It is for a special kind of loving, the kind that is creative of new beings like ourselves. That is why it will always remain the *mysterium tremendum.* It represents and actualizes the best that is in us.

Homosexual acts necessarily exclude any relation to procreation, even the minimal relation that still exists in contraceptive or sterile heterosexual acts. Homosexual acts exclude in principle any reference to procreation and to that extent they diminish the full meaning of human sexuality.

On the objective level, therefore, homosexuality will never measure up to or adequately reflect the full significance of human sexuality. This is true even of the best homosexual activity, that which is truly expressive of interpersonal love.

On the personal level homosexuality can and frequently does depreciate the meaning of human sexuality in a further way. Often it is not even an expression of love. It is neither life-giving nor lovemaking. In such cases it is simply the selfish taking of venereal pleasure through the use of another person's body and it entails the concomitant depersonalization of the other.

An act of personal intimacy is one thing; biological sex without feeling or caring is quite another. Sexual intercourse is a sign of total, unreserved giving of self. At the moment of orgasm the individual's personality is lost in an interpenetration of the other self. Sexual intercourse is expressive of one's person. To be authentic and not a lie it must correspond to the existing relationship between the persons.

Many homosexual acts, especially those among men, are in fact acts of depersonalized sex. They not only nullify in principle the procreative intent of human sexual love; they also regularly presuppose the absence of all emotional contact and responsible pledge.

In conclusion, then, homosexual acts necessarily exclude all relation to procreation, and they frequently are not more than mechanical, depersonalized acts of self-gratification. Human sexuality is better than that. That is why we cannot simply say that homosexuality is morally neutral, that it makes no difference whether one is homosexual or heterosexual, as if there were no important values or meaning at stake.

The preceding analysis is an attempt to isolate what is morally wrong with homosexuality on the level of ethical theory. It does not say that homosexuality is perverse or rotten or that anyone who engages in it is evil. It only says that it devalues the meaning of human sexuality in at least one and frequently two significant ways.

Each of us finds his place somewhere on a homosexual-heterosexual continuum. Some people are exclusively heterosexual; some, exclusively homosexual; and the rest, somewhere in between. A scale of one to seven would include the following classifications: (1) exclusively heterosexual; (2) predominantly heterosexual, but incidentally homosexual; (3) predominantly heterosexual, but more than incidentally homosexual; (4) equally heterosexual and homosexual; (5) predominantly homosexual, but more than incidentally heterosexual; (6) predominantly homosexual, but incidentally heterosexual; and (7) exclusively homosexual.

Individuals can be located on this continuum according to either their psychic response or their actual behavior.

In most cases overt behavior will follow psychic response, but in some instances actual behavior will differ from psychic response. For instance, an inmate in a penitentiary or a boy in a military academy might be classified as predominantly heterosexual according to psychic response, but predominantly homosexual according to actual behavior. One's psychic response, of course, is the more important factor, and except in unusual circumstances it will determine one's overt behavior.[6]

One cannot rule out the possibility that even a person who is exclusively homosexual can change sufficiently to live a normal heterosexual life. This is especially true if the homosexual is highly motivated. But there is only a very small likelihood of this happening. In fact, there is only a small likelihood of substantial change by anyone whose psychic response has been either exclusively homosexual or predominantly homosexual and only incidentally heterosexual for a period of five to ten years. This does not imply that therapy has no value, only that it has limited value. Whenever possible it should be tried. Sometimes it will succeed at least in some useful degree. But more frequently it will fail, and nothing more can be done.

It should be noted that while the homosexual frequently is not free in determining his basic psychic response, he is usually free and in control of his actual behavior. His homosexual acts are not compulsive acts. Normally he has the same degree of personal control over his overt sexual behavior as a heterosexual person has over his.

One should try first of all to ascertain what exactly someone means when he says that he is homosexual. Is he exclusively or almost exclusively homosexual in his psychic needs and response? Or is he able to switch? If he is able to behave heterosexually, then he ought to. It is not enough for him simply to say that gay is good and to behave as if homosexuality were a morally indifferent matter. To freely choose homosexuality as a way of life when it is possible to do otherwise is a serious depreciation and mockery of the full human and Christian meaning of sex.

Second, if someone cannot behave heterosexually, then ordinarily he ought to try to get some professional help. Therapy may or may not be useful, but usually it will be worth a try. In normal circumstances therapy would be ordinary means to protect some very important values. Therapy usually will require the homosexual to engage in physical intimacies with persons of the opposite sex, and I think that in the circumstances one could counsel this as the lesser evil.

But what if there is no way that a person can change? What if he is irreformably homosexual in his psychic response and needs? This is the most difficult question, and it is being addressed in the theological literature in a very halting and exploratory way. The theological analysis of this question is far from complete, and it appears that no significant consensus has yet been reached.

One tentative solution is that a confirmed homosexual may choose the lesser of two evils—namely, a permanent homosexual relationship built on mutual love rather than a life of casual promiscuity. The homosexual may do this only because heterosexuality is impossible and celibacy is not a truly viable option. Therefore, the lesser evil is the only possible good in the circumstances.[7]

The weakness in this analysis is that it does not provide any solution for the many homosexuals who are unable to establish a permanent homosexual relationship built on mutual love and whose only choice therefore is between celibacy and casual promiscuity.

Another solution, based on the principle of compromise, asserts that because of the presence of sin and its effects in the world, homosexuality would not be objectively wrong in those circumstances in which it is the only viable alternative for an individual. Homosexual behavior will never be the ideal, but it can be reluctantly accepted as the only possible good when it is the only way an individual can find a satisfying degree of humanity in his life.[8]

It seems to me that this solution is acceptable as a practical norm, but that there is a certain haziness in the theoretical principle that grounds it. I would suggest a somewhat different rationale which is a bit more precise and comes to the same practical conclusion. It is based on Schüller's preference-principle as refined by Josef Fuchs. The principle states that premoral evil becomes moral evil only when done without a proportionate reason. Homosexual acts in themselves represent human disvalues in a premoral sense. They become moral evil in those circumstances in which there is no proportionate reason for doing them. But if there is a proportionate reason for such acts, they remain premoral disvalues and not immoral even on the objective level. I would think that very often an individual's inability ever to engage in normal heterosexual acts would count as such a proportionate reason.

CHAPTER **6**

GENETIC MANIPULATION

It is by now widely known that the life sciences, especially the recent discoveries in molecular biology, have made possible the redoing of the human race. Until 1944 the life sciences provided only qualitative descriptions. They were not one of the exact sciences, like physics or chemistry, which used precise measurements that could lay the basis for confident predictions and mechanical manipulations. The breakthrough in the life sciences comparable to the breakthroughs in physics by Galileo and Newton and in chemistry by Lavoisier came in 1944 when Oswald T. Avery and two associates at the Rockefeller Institute discovered the properties of a substance called deoxyribonucleic acid (DNA). Experiments by James D. Watson and Francis Crick in 1953 confirmed that DNA is the "secret of life." Hidden in the spiral-staircase structure of this, the master molecule of life, are the mysteries of heredity, growth, aging, disease, and perhaps even memory and intelligence.[1]

The recent discoveries of molecular biology have given man enormous power over human life. He has the scientific knowledge to enable him to radically manipulate and refashion the human species. All that is necessary is the development of certain technological skills. Some of the necessary techniques are already available. The others will be developed in time.

In the past technology has been able to harness and make general use of scientific breakthroughs within about sixty years. For instance, within sixty years Oersted's accidental discovery of the connection between electricity and magnetism in 1820 had been channeled by technology into electrical generators and motors, the telegraph, the incandescent light, and the electrification of the world. The "edison effect" first discovered by Thomas Edison in 1883 gave birth to the science of electronics and within sixty years had been put to use in the production of radios, televisions, and gigantic computers. Becquerel's observation in 1896 of certain properties of uranium made it possible within fifty years for scientists to smash atoms and atoms to smash cities. In 1926 Goddard sent the first rocket powered with liquid fuel and liquid oxygen 184 feet in the air at a speed of sixty miles an hour; within thirty-five years technological advances enabled us to put men into orbit around the earth, and within fifty years, to land men on the moon.[2]

The possibilities laid open by the cracking of the genetic code and by other recent discoveries in the life sciences already have been widely publicized. Artificial insemination of human beings has been going on since 1884.[3] It is estimated that about one hundred and fifty thousand people in the United States were conceived through artificial insemination and that ten thousand people are born each year through such conception. Frozen sperm will enable men to generate sons and daughters long after their own deaths. The sperm is mixed with glycerol, sealed in a bottle, and frozen in liquid nitrogen at a temperature of −324°F. When needed it is thawed and injected into the uterus. According to a 1971 report in *Newsweek,* Dr. Edward T. Tyler of Los Angeles already had enabled sixty-eight women to have babies by means of artificial insemination with sperm frozen for as long as 2½ years.

Artificial inovulation is already feasible in humans. An ovum taken directly from the ovaries is fertilized in a test tube and the zygote is reimplanted in the uterus. Or the zygote can be implanted in the uterus of another woman who will carry it through the gestation period and bring the child to birth. (One fanciful account pictures a woman strolling through a special kind of market selecting frozen embryos guaranteed free from all genetic defects and described on the labels as to sex, eye color, probable I.Q., and so on. The embryo selected can be brought home, thawed out, and implanted by a physician.) After the perfection of an artificial placenta, another option will be ectogenesis, gestation in an artificial womb.

Asexual reproduction also is on the horizon and will probably be practicable in human beings before the end of the present century. It already has been successfully achieved in lower animals. One method is by nuclear transplantation, or cloning.[4] The nucleus of an unfertilized ovum will be destroyed by ultraviolet radiation and then replaced by the nucleus of a cell taken from the body of some other person. The ovum then will have a full set of chromosomes and so will begin to divide as if it had been fertilized; eventually it will develop into the identical twin of the person who supplied the nucleus for the transplant. In this way it will be possible to make exact copies or replicas of any human being. No sexual activity will be involved, and there will be no admixture of the chromosomal material or genetic information of a second person in the newly xeroxed human being. This process of producing clones of genetically identical individuals has already been successful with tadpoles and frogs. The technical problems involved in doing the same thing for humans should be solved before the end of this century.

The possibilities are intriguing. Carbon copies could be made of such men and women as Linus Pauling, Wernher von Braun, Simon and Garfunkel, Henry Kissinger, Joe

Namath, Ann-Margret, Raquel Welch, Dan Berrigan, Johnny Carson, or yourself. By a process of "clonal farming" people could provide for themselves genetically identical spare organs or parts in case an organ transplant ever became necessary.

The creation of animal-human chimeras is also expected. This will be accomplished by introducing certain nonhuman genetic material into developing human embryos or human genetic material into developing subhuman embryos. Thus a new species of parahumans will be created to be used in servile jobs. The mixture of animals and plants and the production of cyborgs, combinations of man and machine, also will be possible.

Gordon Taylor draws out some of the social implications of creating chimeras: "What will be the legal status of a creature with human chromosomes but animal appearance? And conversely? Human nature being what it is, men will be more horrified at the killing of a creature which looks like a man but is not, than when the reverse combination is the victim, though reason would suggest the opposite. How shall we define man? How man-like need one be to qualify for human benefits, including access to the retirement pension or to union membership? It is not fantasy to say that in our lifetime unions may be faced with competition from intelligent apes, which may make British coal-miners' objection to Polish miners, and American racial difficulties, look like child's play."[5]

Genetic surgery (micro- or nano-surgery) also may be practiced before the end of this century. It will be possible to correct genetic defects by the removal of mutant genes or the introduction of normal genes either transplanted from other organisms or synthesized chemically. Man as he now exists will be reengineered: he could be genetically programmed, for instance, to grow an extra thumb for more efficient hands, develop protruding eyes for better peripheral vision, develop a larger brain, or acquire the power to regenerate organs like the lungs or heart. Once technology has caught up with science, man will be able to take hold of his own evolution and to develop himself in whatever direction he thinks best.

It is easy to see that scientific progress is not all that hangs in the balance here. Some basic human values are at stake. Francis Crick has remarked that "there is going to be no agreement between Christians and any humanists who lack their particular prejudice about the sanctity of the individual, and who simply want to try it scientifically."[6] Another American scientist has anonymously stated that "if I can carry a baby all the way through to birth in vitro, I certainly plan to do it—although, obviously I'm not going to succeed on the first attempt or even the twentieth."[7] Discussing the moral concerns of the church, Francois Houtart argues that "the problem of tomorrow is the control of genetics."[8] Richard McCormick observes that "if genetics is the problem of tomorrow, it is already the problem of today if we are to wrest from technology the dictation of policy in this vitally important sphere."[9]

The church does not need another Galileo case. Neither does she need to rush in to baptize whatever is scientifically and technologically possible. That something is technologically possible does not mean that it is therefore desirable or that man ought to do it. Man has uncovered secrets that will allow him to produce human beings in test tubes, control human evolution, and alter the species. Entering on this course will be the most fateful act in his history. What is more, profound human and religious values are involved, among them marriage and the family, parenthood, human life, and freedom. These values are certain to be challenged by the new embryologists. The decision cannot go to science and technology by default. Man must decide, and so the Christian is forced to reexamine his traditional values in the light of the Gospel as well as in the light of the new possibilities now laid open for mankind. James Gustafson has stated the issue for Christians: "Are there limits to man's tampering with human life which have a . . . direct relationship to religious beliefs?"[10]

Artificial Insemination

According to Helmut Thielicke, "the borderline situations which compel us to seek the whys and wherefores" are the "truly propitious places for acquiring knowledge."[11] AID (artificial insemination by a donor) is such a borderline. A consideration of it will sort out at the start one of the fundamental ethical issues inherent in the eugenic proposals of the revolutionary biologists.

Eugenic proposals for the improvement of the human race are not new. The possibilities of eugenic sterilization and donar insemination have been with us for a long time. Gordon Taylor reminds us that a eugenic program was suggested by Plato when he had Socrates say, "If we want to prevent the human race degenerating, we shall take care to encourage union between the better specimens of both sexes and to limit the worse." At the end of the nineteenth century a group of English eugenicists led by Galton stimulated renewed interest in the planned breeding of men, and Adolph Hitler actually put a limited eugenic program into practice in Nazi Germany.

There are two ways in which planned breeding can be practiced. One is called negative eugenics; the other, positive eugenics. Negative eugenics attempts to breed out bad genes by limiting or terminating reproduction by individuals carrying bad genes. This can be done by genetic counseling, legal prohibition, or voluntary or involuntary sterilization. Positive eugenics tries to breed in good or superior genes by the preferential breeding of superior individuals in the same way that animal breeders breed superior stock.

Because these techniques have clashed with certain traditional values, they have never been seriously considered by most men. What forces us to consider them more seriously now is the predicted genetic future of the human race. There is a divergence of scientific opinion about man's genetic future, but it is generally acknowledged that there is a problem, and most scientists view the outcome pessimistically. Many believe that unless man takes hold of his genetic future, the inevitable prognosis is for the extinction of the human species.

Paul Ramsey reports the predictions of the late Nobel Prize winner, Herman J. Müller.[12] According to Müller and his school of geneticists, if the human race is to survive we must control the quality as well as the quantity of our human population. Euphenics (the science and art of improving or correcting the defects and illnesses of people without affecting their genes) makes its advances at the expense of eugenics. The more progress man makes in correcting defects in the phenotype, the greater the burden of bad genes the race must bear. For by correcting or preventing the expression of detrimental genes, euphenics permits the survival of the biologically unfit, and the biologically unfit continue to procreate more like themselves. Therefore, what is good for the individual and the generation now alive is bad for the human race. For instance, such genetic defects as myopia, diabetes, and mental retardation will continue to spread and increase in the human race for as long as medical science keeps people with these defects alive and able to procreate more of the same. In addition to the load of genetic defects received from previous generations, 20 percent of the present generation suffer new, deleterious mutations. Therefore, just to keep the race at the present level, 20 percent of us will have to become genetically extinct.

Because of the continuing advances of euphenics and the continuing deleterious genetic mutations, the genetic load carried by the human race will finally crush it. According to Müller, within a few million years human beings will be a lot of "hopeless utterly diverse genetic monstrosities." All of society's efforts will be consumed in simply ministering to infirmities. Everyone will be an invalid and will have to exhaust his energies simply in staying alive. This hospital civilization will finally break down—especially since the doctors will be subject to the same genetic deterioration—and man will not be saved from his own biological corruption. So the human race will end, not with a bang but a whimper.

Ramsey focuses the ethical question from the point of view of a Christian. He points out that when a Christian hears Müller's gloomy prediction that a time will come when there will be no more like us to come after us, he will have to reply that he knew this all along. The Christian apocalypse described in the Book of Revelation, Mark 13, and parallel passages gives us the same news in other rhetoric. The idea that we are made out of genes and unto genes we shall return is consonant with the Christian belief that God means to kill us all in the end.

This does not imply that the Christian will do nothing or will be fatalistically unconcerned about genetic deterioration and extinction of the human race. But it does mean, Ramsey says, that as he goes about the urgent business of preventing this calamity, he knows that he is not obliged by any absolute command of God to succeed in his endeavor. He is not bound to succeed in preventing the extinction of the race through genetic deterioration any more than he is bound to prevent planets from colliding with the earth or the cooling of the sun, especially since success is not promised to him by either Scripture or sound reason.

In other words, the Christian knows that he is not bound to succeed at any cost. He knows that he cannot deduce his obligations from some absolutely imperative end without any reference to an ethic of means. In discharging his obligation to future generations, he also is obliged not to dehumanize the present generation of men. Thielicke's remark that an "act of compassion to one generation can be an act of oppression to the next" cuts both ways.

In order to avoid the genetic cul-de-sac into which the human race is heading, Müller proposes that we begin a system of breeding human beings toward a desired genotype. Attempts at negative eugenics—breeding out bad genes—offer little hope of gain for the human race because the bad genes will be preserved as recessives in great numbers in heterozygotes like man. What is needed now, Müller says, is the establishment of deep-frozen sperm banks with detailed records of the life and health of the phenotype donor. Donors should be selected from among the outstanding men of our time, and a campaign of education and propaganda should be launched so that in twenty years most women will freely choose to be inseminated by the sperm of one of these intellectual, emotional, or moral geniuses.

Quickly passing over the scientific and sociopsychological objections that might be raised against this plan, Ramsey moves straight to a moral problem that rises in Christian ethics.[13] The Christian understanding of human sexuality is not based on natural law in the sense that it is derived from a reflection on biological function. Rather it is based on the Christian story of creation which is found not in the Book of Genesis but in the Prologue of the Gospel of John and Ephesians 5. Here we learn that God created everything out of his love: God's love is creative. Human love is made in the image of God's love; hence human love is procreative. God's love is normative for human love. Therefore, we may not separate in principle our love and our procreation. That is to say, we may not separate the spheres of personal love and procreation. This does not mean that each individual act of love must be procreative; it does not mean that contraception is immoral. But it does mean that fornication and AID are immoral—fornication because it separates the sphere of personal love from the sphere of responsible procreation and AID because it separates the sphere of procreation from the sphere of personal love. To separate the two is "a refusal of the image of God's creation in our own."

In Ramsey's view, what is at stake is the Christian meaning of love and parenthood. This, of course, can be questioned. Is not conception through AID merely a kind of preadoption? Is not an adopted child also the fruit of love? Michael Hamilton puts it this way: "Parenthood in its deepest sense is not a biological but a *human* function—of a man and wife accepting responsibility for caring for and rearing a child. . . . I believe that the demand of love in relation to parenthood is fulfilled in ensuring that all children born into this world, by whatever means, be reared in a family."[14]

Commenting on Hamilton's contribution, McCormick observes that limiting the notion of love and parenthood to caring for and rearing a child is a "radical attack on several basic humano-Christian values (the meaning of human sexuality, the meaning of marriage and parenthood)."[15] In the Christian perspective the parental love that nurtures is an extension or continuation of the sexual love that generates: parents do not love their children simply because they are there and in need of love; they love them because they are the fruit of their love for one another. Besides, McCormick argues, Hamilton's distinction between a merely biological function and a human function reflects a dualistic anthropology. Men love and care not only with their minds but with their bodies, with their sexuality. The biological function of sexual intercourse is not separable from but is the human function of loving.

At the present stage of the debate I think it is fair to say that the arguments of Ramsey and McCormick are persuasive. They do not, however, close the question beyond doubt. They provide a satisfactory rationale for our traditional understanding of sexuality, marriage, and parenthood. This understanding reflects human values which run deep and have been with us for a long time. It would be next to impossible, or at least extremely difficult, ever to change them. But I do not think that the arguments have the decisive cogency that Ramsey seems to attribute to them. A more modest and sensible conclusion is reached by Charles Curran: "I do believe that at the present time in our circumstances sexuality has its proper expression, value and meaning in the marital realm within which the procreative and love union aspects of sexuality are joined together. However, one can envision a possibility in which greater values might be at stake and call for some type of altering the way in which Christian marriage now tries to preserve these important values. For example, if the dire predictions of Müller were universally accepted and mankind did face a genetic apocalypse in the near future, then the entire situation might be changed. It seems that even the Scriptures witness many cases in which the understanding of marriage had to be changed because of the conditions of the times (e.g. polygamy). . . . I agree with Ramsey's understanding of things as they are at present, but his argumentation and his prospect in the future do not seem to give enough place to historicity."[16]

The Magisterium

On 24 March 1897 the question was put to the Holy Office: Can artificial fecundation of a woman be used? The answer: It is not permitted.[17] This reply was approved and confirmed by the Holy Father.

One of the issues scarcely hidden here was masturbation.

Masturbation, judged intrinsically evil, was the obvious means of procuring semen. If semen could be collected in some licit way, would artificial insemination be permitted at least when the woman's husband was the donor (AIH)? A good number of reputable Catholic moralists thought so. They argued that semen could be procured licitly by aspiration from the epididymis or testicles, by aspiration from the vagina after normal intercourse, or by using a perforated condom during intercourse. If semen were gathered in one of these licit ways, they reasoned, at least AIH would be moral.

The theologians had opened a doorway leading to at least some form of artificial insemination. That door was promptly closed by Pope Pius XII. Addressing the Fourth International Convention of Catholic Physicians on 29 September 1949, he said that artificial insemination is to be "absolutely rejected." He stated that "artificial insemination outside marriage is to be condemned purely and simply as immoral" and that "artificial insemination within marriage, with the use of an active element from a third person, is equally immoral and as such to be rejected summarily."[18] He added in explanation that the marriage contract does not confer upon couples any right to use artificial insemination, since "the contract has as its object not a child but the natural acts apt and destined for the generation of new life."[19] Theologians generally read this explanation as excluding AIH.

If there was any doubt, the pope clarified his position two years later in his address to the Congress of the Italian Catholic Union of Midwives on 26 November 1951, when he said: "To reduce the cohabitation of married persons and the conjugal act to a mere organic function for the transmission of the germ of life would be to convert the domestic hearth, sanctuary of the family, into nothing more than a biological laboratory. Hence in our address of

September 29, 1949, to the international congress of Catholic doctors, we formally excluded artificial insemination from marriage. The conjugal act in its natural structure is a personal action, a simultaneous mutual self-giving which, in the words of Holy Scripture, effects the union 'in one flesh.' This is much more than the mere union of two germs, which can be brought about also artificially, that is, without the natural action of the spouses. The conjugal act, as it is planned and willed by nature, implies a personal cooperation, the right to which the partners have mutually conferred on each other in contracting marriage."[20]

Theologians picked up the pope's central argument. In God's design human love is procreative. Man must not put asunder what God has joined together. As it is wrong to separate procreation from the act of sexual love in contraception, it is equally wrong to separate the act of sexual love from procreation in artificial insemination (AID and AIH).

The difference between the pope's argument and Ramsey's is that the pope thought that the procreative and unitive aspects of human sexuality may not be separated even in an individual act, whereas Ramsey only objects to their separation in principle, i.e., the separation of the spheres of love and procreation. Ramsey therefore concludes to the immorality of only AID, not AIH. Obviously, one who admits exceptions to papal teaching on contraception ought logically to admit exceptions to papal teaching on AIH, for these teachings are of a piece.

Richard McCormick accepts the pope's teaching on AIH as generally true. If procreation ordinarily were to be achieved among men through AIH, then we "would have taken a long step toward biologizing and mechanizing marriage." Human love is meant to be procreative and the child is meant to be the fruit of this love. Therefore it is certainly wrong to routinely use AIH in place of natural intercourse if it is not required. But if a couple having sexual relations remains sterile, it is not at all clear that the use of AIH would necessarily turn marriage into a biological laboratory. McCormick therefore suggests that the papal statements may be closer to law than teaching and that it is "possible to admit the licitness of the exceptional instance."[21]

Today a good number of Catholic moralists would find no objection to a childless couple's using AIH even when the semen is obtained by masturbation. Commenting on Roger Van Allen's defense of this procedure,[22] Robert Springer says, "Recent moral analysis is disinclined to view the external action by which the semen is obtained as constituting the moral entity of the act."[23] That is to say, masturbation that is necessary for the artificial insemination of one's wife or for semen analysis cannot be morally evaluated simply as a physical or biological act. It receives its moral significance and specification from the purposes and circumstances of the agent.

Some Tentative Casuistry

With the foregoing as background it may be useful to engage in some casuistry. What I propose to do is to sort out a few concrete issues, offer a tentative judgment, and indicate the reasons for that judgment. That the opinions at this stage are tentative should come as no surprise. As Harmon Smith has pointed out, in this area an unwillingness to be definitive is not the same as an inability to be decisive; it only reflects an awareness of one's limited understanding of all that may be involved in some very complex issues that are facing us for the first time in human history.

Generally speaking, reproduction of human beings by any method other than normal sexual intercourse would seem to be opposed to the human and Christian meaning of man's sexuality and parenthood. As Ramsey points out, man is the body of his soul as well as the soul of his body, and it is through his bodily sexuality that he realizes his human power to love and create other beings like himself. To separate in principle the realm of human love from the realm of human procreation is to refuse the image of God's creative love in human procreative loving. Therefore, attempts to breed a new or super race of men through a system of frozen sperm banks and AID would strike very deeply at the *humanum* in man.

However, if the predictions of Müller were proven, another conclusion might be reached. Pursuant to Schüller's preference-principle, one ought to prefer the radical redefinition of the human race to its total extinction. I share Charles Curran's view that "parenthood and family bonds are more than antiquated traditions. For the Christian, the bond between procreation and love union is more than a mere arbitrary arrangement even if one can envision certain historical situations in which it might be sacrificed for greater values."[24]

I also think that AIH generally should be excluded unless it is the only way an otherwise sterile couple can achieve procreation. If in particular cases it is required for procreation, masturbation would seem to be a morally acceptable technique of obtaining sperm from the husband, since the moral meaning of the physical act is derived from the circumstances and purpose toward which it is directed.

Artificial inovulation runs into the same problem as artificial insemination. To create new beings like ourselves in laboratory test tubes rather than in the midst of our love for one another would constitute a radical shift away from the humano-Christian understanding of man's life-giving love. I would not, however, want to rule out absolutely every instance. Artificial inovulation might be tolerable or even morally the better option in certain circumstances —for instance, if the only way a woman can conceive a child is through the fertilization of one of her ova by her husband's sperm in a test tube and the implantation of the fertilized ovum in her uterus for gestation.[25] Perhaps in this extraordinary case test-tube fertilization would not undermine or clash with the Christian understanding of man's life-giving love but could be interpreted as an effort to measure up fully to that understanding in the only way possible. In such special circumstances the technical procedure of fertilization would be the only way to allow the couple's genuine sharing of human sexual love to come to its normal fruition in a child.

The same judgment could be made even if it were necessary to implant the conceptus in the uterus of another woman or to put it in an artificial womb in order to bring it through the gestation period to maturity. A practical problem would have to be carefully weighed: Would the implantation of the conceptus in the womb of another woman who would bring the child to birth create disproportionate emotional problems for either the real or the host mother? A practical decision would depend largely on the temperament and emotional makeup of the women involved.

Nuclear transplantation or cloning also represents a radical assault on the meaning of conjugal intercourse as a life-giving act of lovemaking and a lovemaking act of life-giving. It would represent a fundamental shift from the human meaning of parenthood, in which the one flesh of the child comes from the one-flesh unity of man and wife together. In addition, a shift to clonal reproduction would in all likelihood be a fatal step backward for the human species. Joshua Lederberg says that "clonality as a way of life in the plant world is well understood as an evolutionary cul-de-sac."[26] If cloning were to replace sexual reproduction, with the result that the population would be distributed not among unique individuals but among millions of clones, man's variability and adaptability would probably be lost, and the human race would lose the very qualities that best insure survival. On the other hand, selective cloning of certain individuals for specialized functions or in order to copy the genotype of certain superior individuals would hardly seem to provide sufficient benefit to justify creating new beings like ourselves apart from our human, life-giving love.

Genetic surgery presents no moral problems in itself. It provides the greatest hope for the future of man. All that is necessary is that the norms commonly observed in all surgery be followed. Specifically, the risk of harm must be proportionate to the hope of benefit for the individual. The risk must be proportionate to the hope of benefit *for the individual*, not for the future of science. Human monstrosities should not be created in order to advance medical knowledge.

Reengineering man presents no inherent moral problems. In fact, Karl Rahner argues that "man is essentially a freedom event." He is created unfinished by God. In his freedom he determines what he will be irrevocably for all eternity. On this earth he should take hold of himself in his freedom and may, if he chooses, modify himself in the innermost depths of his biological, genetic, psychological, and historical existence.[27]

Rahner's analysis is quite correct in theory, and that is why I say that reengineering man presents no inherent moral problems. But practically speaking man needs not only science, technology, and the will to alter the species —he also needs the wisdom necessary to do it to the benefit and not the destruction of the species. I do not see evidence of this sort of wisdom in man at this moment. Dr. J. Russell Elkinton, editor of the *Annals of Internal Medicine*, is quoted in the *New York Times* (28 March 1971) as saying: "What man can do is becoming more obvious. What man ought to do is yet a dark enigma." There are two factors that make it appear questionable that man presently has enough wisdom to remake man. The first is that there are too many unknown variables for us to set long-range goals for the human race as a whole. Genes that are considered bad now may become necessary in the event of environmental change, and variability and flexibility have always been the most important assets in a species' struggle for survival. The second problem that must be better resolved is one of values. What traits are in fact genetically good and what traits are bad in the race? Who will decide what man should be like, and according to what standards? Genetic imprudence now could be a very costly if not fatal mistake for the human race. Charles Curran once remarked that "if we are going to do something like this to the species, someone is going to have to decide and plan what sort of men we ought to become, and if the genetic planners are anything like those who have been planning our domestic and foreign policies, God help us."

On the question of chimeras and cyborgs, I simply do not know what to say, mainly because I do not understand what these creatures are to be. If they are to be superior animals and machines created by the introduction of human genetic material into developing subhuman embryos, perhaps we should make them. But if they are to be inferior or subhuman men created by the introduction of nonhuman genetic material into developing human embryos, it would be wicked to make them.

A final caution: in thinking about questions such as these we must be on guard against naiveté and one-sided optimism. Sacred Scripture reminds us that there is a principle of evil abroad. H. Richard Niebuhr has wisely cautioned against a liberalism that is naively optimistic, that would have us believe that "a God without wrath brought men without sin into a kingdom without judgment through the ministrations of a Christ without a cross."[28] In our enthusiasm and hope for the future, it would be unwise to forget that man has been, is, and always will be sinful man. Of course he must play God—there is no other way. But he is not God, and given the role without surveillance and control, he can become a devil.

C. S. Lewis has observed that man's power over nature is really the power of some men over other men, with nature their instrument. It is not so much the evil scientist that we must fear as the capacity for evil in every man. As P. B. Medawar has said: "The Wicked Scientist is not to be taken seriously: Dr. Strangelove, Dr. Moreau, Dr. Moriarty, Dr. Mabuse, Dr. Frankenstein (an honorary degree, this) and the rest of them are puppets of Gothic fiction. Scientists, on the whole, are amiable and well-meaning creatures. There must be very few wicked scientists. There are, however, plenty of wicked philosophers, wicked priests, and wicked politicians."[29] Such men are capable of the gravest mischief.

Part Three

Human Life

CHAPTER 7

ABORTION

In the Greco-Roman world in which Christianity arose, abortion was widely practiced, especially among the upper classes, in spite of some opposition from philosophers, physicians, and legislators. Plato had accepted abortion for population control and so had Aristotle, but only before "sensation and life." The gynecologist Soranos of Ephesus (A.D. 98-138) opposed it except when the life of the mother was endangered, and physicians taking the Hippocratic oath swore: "I will not give to a woman an abortifacient pessary." Roman law prohibited giving abortifacient drugs which were dangerous to the mother and forbade any abortion not done with the father's consent. But all the opposition had little practical influence on those who wanted an abortion for personal advantage.

The New Testament, like the Old, contains no clear condemnation of abortion.[1] *Pharmakeia,* the magical practice of medicine by "medicine men," was condemned (Gal. 5:20; Apoc. 9:21, 21:8, 20:15), and this condemnation no doubt included the giving of magical potions and drugs to induce an abortion. But abortion as such is not mentioned in the Bible.

The first clear repudiation of abortion in Christian literature appears in the *Didache,* which was written in about A.D. 100: "You shall not kill. You shall not commit adultery. You shall not corrupt boys. You shall not fornicate. You shall not steal. You shall not make magic. You shall not practice medicine [*pharmakeia*]. You shall not slay the child by abortions. You shall not kill what is generated. You shall not desire your neighbor's wife."

The word used for abortion here is *phthorion,* which had been expressly distinguished by Soranos from *ekbolion:* it meant "destroying what has been conceived" as distinguished from "expelling what has been conceived."

The *Epistle of Barnabas* (ca. 117-31) put the *Didache's* prohibition of abortion in the context of the command to love one's neighbor: "You shall love your neighbor more than your own life. You shall not slay the child by abortions. You shall not kill what is generated." And the *Apocalypse of Peter* (ca. 150) says that in the pit of torment are women "who have caused their children to be born untimely and have corrupted the work of God who created them."

Early church fathers like Clement of Alexandria, Minucius Felix, Cyprian, Tertullian, Jerome, Augustine, Basil, and John Chrysostom repeated this general condemnation of abortion. The Council of Ancyra (314) condemned abortion but reduced the penalty for women who aborted an illegitimate child from lifetime excommunication to ten years, and in the years between five hundred and eleven hundred local synods reiterated the canons of Ancyra.

The early Fathers condemned abortion in general and were especially concerned about abortions performed in connection with fornication and adultery. But only Tertullian discussed the problem of therapeutic abortion performed to save the life of the mother. Like the other Fathers he was an antiabortionist, and he defended intrauterine life as fully human: "But for us, to whom murder has been once for all forbidden, it is not permitted to destroy even what has been conceived, while as yet the blood is still being formed into a human being. Interruption of a pregnancy is a hastening of murder, and it makes no difference whether it is a soul already born that is snatched away or a soul in process of being born that is interfered with. He is a human being who will be one; the whole fruit is actually in the seed."[2] But concerning the special case of an abortion that is necessary to save the life of the mother he wrote: "But sometimes by cruel necessity, while yet in the womb, an infant is put to death, when lying awry in the orifice of the womb he impedes parturition, and kills his mother, if he is not to die himself."[3]

In the early Middle Ages theologians and canonists discussed the question of the time of ensoulment: At what point does God infuse the rational soul into the newly conceived body? But the question, originally raised by Jerome and Augustine, was of more speculative than practical interest to them. Even though many believed that ensoulment does not take place until after the body reaches a certain stage of development and that abortion before ensoulment is not homicide, they agreed that abortion before ensoulment is wrong because it has at least the malice of contraception.

Between the fifteenth and the eighteenth centuries some theologians began to allow the abortion of a nonanimated fetus to save the life of the mother.[4] Pope Sixtus V in 1588 and Pope Gregory XIV in 1591 condemned contraception and the abortion of animated and nonanimated fetuses.[5] But both popes spoke in general terms about abortion and were directly concerned with the abortions connected with prostitution in Rome. Neither pope mentioned anything about therapeutic abortion, and so their decrees had no influence on the teaching of the more lenient moralists of the time.

The Holy See remained quiet on the matter for another

century. Then in 1679 Innocent XI condemned sixty-five lax moral opinions. Two of these had to do with abortion: (1) it is licit to procure an abortion before the animation of the fetus so that a girl who is discovered pregnant will not be killed or defamed; and (2) it seems probable that every fetus (as long as it is in the uterus) lacks a rational soul and first begins to have one when it is born; and therefore it must be said that no homicide is committed in abortion.[6] These propositions were condemned as "at least scandalous and in practice dangerous."

Contemporary Catholic Teaching

The official contemporary teaching of the Catholic Church took final shape near the end of the nineteenth and at the beginning of the twentieth century. One of the principal antagonists was the outstanding moralist of the time, Augustine Lehmkuhl, S. J. One can trace the development of the struggle between him and Rome in the various editions of his *Theologia Moralis*. In the earlier editions he also describes the developing theological scene that brought the Holy See into action.[7]

Many of the earlier authors had defended embryotomy before ensoulment in order to save the life of the mother. Their principal argument was that the fetus was a materially unjust aggressor against the mother's life and that therefore she had the right to defend herself by killing the fetus, just as one has the right to kill a madman attacking him, even though the madman is subjectively innocent and not responsible for his action.

But if the fetus was to be considered an involuntary aggressor, why did these authors restrict embryotomy to the time before ensoulment occurred? Was not the animated fetus also a material aggressor? The reason for their restriction was not that the ensouled fetus was a human being but that he was a human being in the state of original sin and so in need of baptism for his eternal salvation. Hence, the older authors reasoned, the eternal life of the fetus took precedence over the temporal life of the mother. They accepted Thomas's opinion that one may not kill the mother in order to baptize the child, but they did not interpret this to mean that one may not and should not await the death of the mother for the same purpose.

Gradually, however, this strict opinion about the obligation of baptism was displaced, and so was Aristotle's biology.[8] The result was that more recent authors no longer attached any importance to the distinction between an animated and a nonanimated fetus. As far as baptism was concerned, they were content to say that one should try to provide for it insofar as possible, but the mother was not bound to give up her life for that purpose. Hence, Lehmkuhl reports, the modern authors became more consistent: they applied the argument of the materially unjust aggressor to the entire time of fetal life, not just to the earlier stages.

The older authors had described this feticide as indirect killing. They used the category of *indirect* in the same sense as Thomas did when he described the killing of an unjust aggressor: one's direct intention is the preservation of one's own life, and the death of the attacker occurs *per accidens* since it is not the direct object of one's intention.[9] Accordingly, an effect was considered direct or indirect depending on one's intention rather than on the nature or objective thrust of the action. De Lugo and others had resisted this usage, but other authors continued to understand the categories in their Thomistic sense.

A contemporary of Lehmkuhl, Antonius Ballerini, S. J., carefully distinguished the two senses in which various authors were understanding the distinction between direct and indirect killing. Ballerini defended the Thomistic usage. Therefore, he concluded, one may never directly will or intend the death of a fetus, but if the death of the mother and child are imminent, the mother is not bound to die. He argued, as the Salmanticenses had noted, that more than twenty theologians considered the fetus a materially unjust aggressor whose death, as Thomas had shown, would be indirect, not the direct object of intent. This, he said, was also the opinion of Tertullian, and it probably reflected the commonly accepted rule in the early Church.[10]

On 28 November 1872 the Sacred Penitentiary was asked: Is it ever permitted to perform an operation called a craniotomy or a similar operation which per se directly tends to the killing of an infant in the womb? The case proposed noted that the practice was to baptize the infant in the womb before its head was crushed. The Sacred Penitentiary responded that it had given the case mature consideration and that anyone facing this problem should consult the approved authors, both ancient and modern, and then act prudently.[11] Ballerini observed that the Sacred Penitentiary's unwillingness to decide the case was not surprising, since the case was so difficult and learned theologians had defended both sides.

A short time later the archbishop of Lyons asked the Holy See for a decision on a similar case: Is a craniotomy licit when it is the only way to prevent both mother and child from dying? This time the Holy Office was less diffident than the Sacred Penitentiary had been in the preceding decade. On 28 May 1884 the Holy Office replied that after long and serious reflection it had decided that it cannot safely be taught in Catholic schools that a craniotomy is licit even when without it both mother and child will die and with it at least the mother can be saved. And again, prompted by a series of questions from the archbishop of Cambrai, on 14 August 1889 the Holy Office repeated its decision of 28 May 1884 and added that neither can it safely be taught in Catholic schools that it is licit to perform any surgical operation that directly kills either the fetus or the mother.[12]

Immediately after these decisions had been promulgated, Ballerini called attention to the fact that the Holy Office had not made a decision about which of the conflicting theological opinions was true. It had merely said that one of the opinions—the one that affirmed the lawfulness of craniotomies—could not be safely taught in Catholic schools. This meant that it could not be taught with a safe conscience or without danger of error. One must, of course, employ great caution in a question of such gravity as the taking of human life, but one may say that a doctrine cannot be safely taught without judging it to be certainly false. It is enough to judge that it is improbable or only tenuously probable. However, what is improbable at one time, Ballerini pointed out, can become probable or even certain at another.

Lehmkuhl accepted the decision of the Holy Office more gracefully. Even before the action of the Holy See he had considered the more lenient opinion, which permitted therapeutic craniotomies, only a probable one, perhaps even less probable than the stricter one, although still safe to follow in practice. After the Roman decision he admitted that people still could easily be in good faith on this question since the arguments were elusive and the Holy See itself had been in doubt only a few years before. But from that time on Lehmkuhl defended the position of the Holy Office, arguing that it is not easy to see how one can consider the fetus a material aggressor when it is only exercising its natural right to be born. On the contrary, he said, one may say with equal or better reason that the mother is a material aggressor against the life of the child.

Nevertheless, many authors, including Lehmkuhl and Ballerini, pointed out that a craniotomy is one thing and abortion quite another. If one accepts de Lugo's definition of *direct* and *indirect* rather than Thomas's, it is easy to see a craniotomy as a direct attack on the fetus. But it is equally obvious that an abortion need not entail any such direct attack. It is true that when an immature or nonviable fetus is artificially ejected from the uterus it will certainly die. But the mother does not directly attack it. She simply ceases to conserve its life. A mother, these authors argued, is not bound to conserve the life of the fetus at the cost of her own. Her duty to conserve the life of her child, both before and after birth, is limited. For instance, a mother who is drowning and cannot swim to safety without letting go of her child is not morally obliged to perish with her child in the sea. She may drop the child and swim to safety rather than drown with the baby. In such a situation she does not murder the child, but regretfully permits its unavoidable death.

Therefore, they taught, if without an abortion both mother and child will die, it is better to abort the child and baptize it. One can thus save the temporal life of the mother and better provide for the eternal life of the child. Furthermore, to induce an abortion when the mother's life is seriously threatened is not direct abortion in the theological or moral sense any more than it is direct suicide to relinquish a plank to another after a shipwreck. One can presume that the fetus would renounce any right to remain in the mother's womb in such circumstances, since it would be unreasonable for the child to do otherwise. Remaining in the womb would be useless for the fetus, while by an acceleration of birth its eternal salvation can be better provided for through baptism.

Therefore, they concluded, the principle of double effect has clear application here.[13] The abortion has two equally immediate effects—the saving of the mother and the death of the fetus. One directly intends to save the mother and has a proportionately grave reason for permitting the death of the fetus. The death of the fetus is not the means that saves the mother. It is rather an immediate consequence of the same action that also results in preserving the mother's life.

The Holy Office did not think so. In 1889 the archbishop of Cambrai sent a number of cases to the Holy Office concerning such things as embryotomies, abortions, and the surgical removal of ectopic pregnancies. On August 19 the Holy See replied vaguely, saying that one may not safely teach that it is licit to perform any operation that directly kills either the mother or the fetus[14]. The archbishop of Cambrai then put the question on abortion more directly: If the only way a pregnant woman can save her life is by aborting an immature fetus that will certainly die soon after its removal from the womb, may she permit an abortion to be performed? On 24 July 1895 the Holy Office answered simply and clearly: "Negatively, in accord with the other decrees of May 28, 1884, and August 19, 1889."[15] This reply was confirmed personally by Pope Leo XIII on the next day.

A series of Roman decisions followed. On 4 May 1898 the Holy See decreed that: (1) acceleration of birth is licit for a good reason if the fetus is ordinarily viable; (2) if a woman's pelvis is too constricted for a normal delivery, abortion of a nonviable fetus is illicit, but a Caesarean section may be performed after viability; and (3) an ectopic fetus may be surgically removed if a realistic attempt is made to see that both mother and child will live.[16]

On 20 March 1900 a more specific question on ectopic pregnancies was submitted: Is it ever permitted to remove an immature ectopic fetus prior to six months of gestation? On 5 May 1902 the Holy See replied in the negative, since ordinarily a fetus at that stage is not viable.[17] Unlike the reply of 1898, this response lacked the personal papal approbation. Lehmkuhl and Bouscaren continued to argue that in the case of a tubal pregnancy the removal of a part of the Fallopian tube along with the nonviable fetus is an indirect abortion, for this operation, unlike the shelling of the fetus out of the tube, does not directly attack the fetus but removes a pathological tube, with the indirect consequence of fetal death. A large number of moralists have agreed that this operation is morally the same as the removal of a cancerous womb in a pregnant woman and so have approved it as an indirect abortion. This opinion has never been reproved by the Holy See.

In 1917 the new Code of Canon Law reiterated the previous legislation: anyone who successfully procures an abortion is ipso facto excommunicated, and absolution from the penalty is reserved to the Ordinary of the diocese.

In 1930 Pope Pius XI made a clear summary of the Roman teaching that had emerged and developed during the previous forty-six years. In *Casti Connubii* he wrote: "But another very grave crime is to be noted, Venerable Brethren, which regards the taking of the life of the offspring hidden in the mother's womb. . . As to the 'medical and therapeutic indication' to which, using their own words, we have made reference, Venerable Brethren, however much we may pity the mother whose health and even life is gravely imperiled in the performance of the duty allotted to her by nature, nevertheless what could ever be a sufficient reason for excusing in any way the direct murder of the innocent? This is precisely what we are dealing with here. Whether inflicted upon the mother or upon the child, it is against the precept of God and the law of nature: 'Thou shalt not kill.' The life of each is equally sacred, and no one has the power, not even the public authority, to destroy it. . . . What is asserted in favor of the social and eugenic 'indication' may and must be accepted . . . but to wish to put forward reasons based upon them for the killing of the innocent is unthinkable and contrary to the divine precept promulgated in the words of the Apostle: Evil is not to be done that good may come of it."[18]

During his long pontificate Pope Pius XII repeated frequently in his public addresses the teaching of his predecessor. Speaking to midwives in 1951 he said: "Every human being, even the child in its mother's womb, receives its right to life directly from God, not from its parents, nor from any human society or authority. Therefore, there is no man, no human authority, no science, no 'indication,' whether medical, eugenical, social, economic or moral, that can show or give a valid juridical title for a deliberate and direct disposing of an innocent human life."[19]

The Second Vatican Council made two statements on abortion. In the Pastoral Constitution on the Church in the Modern World (*Gaudium et Spes*), the bishops said: "Whatever is opposed to life itself, such as any type of murder, genocide, abortion, euthanasia, or willful self-destruction . . . all these things and others of their like are infamies indeed."[20] Near the end of the same document they said: "For God, the Lord of Life, has conferred on men the surpassing ministry of safeguarding life—a ministry which must be fulfilled in a manner which is worthy of man. Therefore from the moment of its conception life must be guarded with the greatest care, while abortion and infanticide are unspeakable crimes."[21]

Finally, in *Humanae Vitae* Pope Paul VI said: "We must once again declare that the direct interruption of the generative process already begun, and, above all, directly willed and procured abortion, even if for therapeutic reasons, are to be absolutely excluded as licit means of regulating birth."[22] On 18 November 1974 this same doctrine was reaffirmed by the Sacred Congregation for the Doctrine of the Faith in its *Declaration on Procured Abortion.*

Until the 1960s Protestant Christians echoed the ancient Church's condemnation of abortion. Calvin, for instance, described it as an "inexpiable crime." Protestant writers did not engage in the same kind of casuistry as Catholics, but churches, theologians, and preachers of all traditions condemned it in general terms. Bonhoeffer was typical in describing abortion as "nothing but murder."[23]

Karl Barth has also described abortion as murder. Nonetheless he admits that sometimes it may be permitted, in fact commanded, by God as *ultima ratio*. Exceptions, however, would be rare and limited to situations in which what is at stake is "life against life."[24]

In 1958 the Lambeth Conference affirmed that "the sacredness of life is, in Christian eyes, an absolute which should not be violated." However, it allowed abortion "at the dictate of strict and undeniable medical necessity." Only during the last decade have Protestant Christians generally assumed a more permissive attitude toward induced abortion.

When Does Human Life Begin?

Before turning to the contemporary theological discussion of abortion, it will be useful to consider the nature of fetal life.

In the act of sexual intercourse about three hundred million sperm are deposited in the vagina. If an ovum has been released from the ovary, one of the sperm may reach and fertilize it. The ovum will live for about twenty-four hours; if fertilization does not occur during this period, both ovum and sperm will die. During the first six to eight hours the sperm must be "capacitated" for fertilization by some substance in the uterus or tube. Fertilization usually occurs in the upper part of the Fallopian tube. It is not instantaneous but is a process taking some minutes. The genes of the father are contained in a packet of twenty-three chromosomes in the sperm and the genes of the mother in a packet of twenty-three chromosomes in the ovum. When fertilization occurs these two packets of chromosomes unite to form a brand new genetic package of forty-six chromosomes, the normal number in a human cell. This genetic package or genotype, which is absolutely new in the universe, is called the zygote.

After a day or two the zygote, while moving down the tube to the uterus, begins a process of daily cleavage or mitosis, splitting into two cells the first day, four cells the second day, eight cells the third day, and so on. The newly divided individual cells, called blastomeres, at the end of four or five days form a cluster of cells called the morula.

The morula begins what is called the blastocyst stage. It enters the uterus and starts the process of implantation in the wall of the uterus: one pole of the cluster of cells (the trophoblast) implants itself in the uterus and becomes the placenta; the other pole (the embryoblast) will become the fetus. The trophoblast begins to introduce hormones into the woman's bloodstream to prevent menstruation, which of course would be fatal to the new life. This process of implantation or nidation takes about six days. By the eleventh day after fertilization the process is completed.

After two weeks the zygote has become more complex, is about one-tenth of an inch long, and is now called the embryo. It seems that identical twins are formed sometime up to this point by the mass of cells splitting into two separate lots. Perhaps twinning takes place a short time after this. Some embryologists believe that it frequently takes place at the primitive streak stage which occurs at the beginning of the third week. Recombination of split or twinned cells into one individual probably can occur during this same time. Therefore, although a new unique individual genotype is formed at conception, it is not irreversibly an individual until about the beginning of its third week of life.

The embryo stage lasts until the end of the eighth week. The heart begins pumping in the third or fourth week. All the internal organs are present in rudimentary form by the end of the sixth week. Reflex movements occur by the end of the seventh week. At the end of eight weeks the embryo is about one inch long. It is fairly well formed, with fingers and toes recognizable, and electrical activity in the brain can be detected in an EEG reading. After the eighth week it is called a fetus.

Between the eight and twelfth weeks reflex and spontaneous movements occur; the fetus grows to about 3½ inches, and its brain structure is completed. After the twelfth week an abortion by scraping the inside of the uterus (D and C) is dangerous to the mother. If an abortion is performed after this time, it is done by abdominal surgery or by injecting a saline solution which causes an immature vaginal delivery into the amniotic sac.

"Quickening" (perception of fetal movement by the mother) usually occurs before the sixteenth week. By the twentieth week the fetus weighs about one pound and is technically viable. A fetus delivered after twenty weeks has about a 10 percent chance of survival today, and so its delivery would be classified as premature, not as an abortion. At the end of the twenty-eighth week the fetus weighs about two pounds and its chance of survival outside the womb has increased substantially. Practically speaking, it is considered viable from the twenty-eighth to the fortieth week, when natural birth usually begins.

Those who argue that individual human life begins at the moment of conception find solid support in the teaching of modern genetics. Paul Ramsey says: "Indeed, microgenetics seems to have demonstrated what religion never could; and biological science, to have resolved an ancient theological dispute. The human individual comes into existence first as a minute informational speck, drawn at random from many other minute informational specks his parents possessed out of the common gene pool. This took place at the moment of impregnation. There were, of course, an unimaginable number of combinations of specks on his paternal and maternal chromosomes that did not come to be when they were refused and he began to be. Still (with the single exception of identical twins), no one else in the entire history of the human race has ever had or will ever have exactly the same genotype. Thus it can be said that the individual is whoever he is going to become from the moment of impregnation. Thereafter, his subsequent development may be described as a process of becoming the one he already is. Genetics teaches that we were from the beginning what we essentially still are in every cell and in every human and individual attribute. . . . What is this but to say that we are all fellow fetuses? That from womb to tomb ours is a nascent life? That we are in essence congeners from the beginning?"[25]

The argument from genotype comes to this. At conception a new and unique genetic package comes into being. This genetic package contains potentially everything that the adult person will become. Man's life is a process of becoming. It would be arbitrary to point to any other moment in this process and say that here a human being emerges. A human being is always emerging, and he is emerging from the initial genetic package which is in potency all that he ever will be.

This position is not only reasonable and scientifically founded; it also most effectively protects the inviolability of human life. For as we shall see, if one tries to designate some point other than conception in the human developmental process as the point of inviolability, it is difficult to avoid arbitrariness in assigning that point. If one accepts in principle that a certain degree of development is necessary before inviolability is established, it is possible that the distinction between abortion and infanticide would become blurred and that dangerous discriminations would be made among human beings of varying potentialities.

There are, however, some difficulties that can be raised against this position. For one thing, it gives no weight to the fact that the potentialities in the genotype are conditioned and shaped by its interaction with the environment. A man, the phenotype, is not simply an enlarged or grown-up genotype. One can reasonably argue that a unique human being is not only a product of his genes. He is a product of a genotype in interaction with other things and people. Hominization is a process which is dependent on more than biochemistry, and therefore genetic individuality alone is too narrow a criterion for establishing that one is truly a human being.

What is more, the zygote is not irreversibly an individual until around the end of the second or the beginning of the third week of life. During that time it may split, forming identical twins (or triplets, etc.). And there is evidence that twinned individuals may recombine, forming again a single genotype. The Christian who adopts the position that a human person exists from the moment of conception can explain, of course, that at the moment of twinning God creates another soul for one of the twins and that if recombination takes place, one of the individual human beings dies, even though there is no organic matter that ceases to live. But he must acknowledge that this scientific data considerably weakens his thesis on the beginning of human life. In a footnote to his argument that human life begins at conception, Paul Ramsey admits the point precisely: "The case of identical twins does, however, suggest a significant modification of any 'proof' from genotype. If there is a moment in the development of nascent life subsequent to impregnation and prior to birth (or graduation from Princeton) at which it would be reasonable to believe that an individual human life *begins* to be inviolate, that moment is arguably at the appearance of a 'primitive streak' across the hollow cluster of developing cells that signals the separation of the same genotype into identical twins."[26]

Other moments in the developmental process have also been suggested as the point of inviolability. One rests on the premise that the existence of a functioning human brain is required for the existence of a human person. Electrical activity in the embryo's developing brain does not start until the eighth week, and the cerebral cortex is not fully complexified until around the sixth month of gestation.

If one takes the appearance of electrical activity in the brain of the embryo as signaling its inviolability, then one has a criterion for judging the beginning of human life that is consistent with the now commonly accepted criterion of death. In 1968, when the possibility of heart transplants had made an exact definition of death more urgent, both a statement of the World Medical Association and a report of an ad hoc committee of the Harvard Medical School agreed that death should be defined as an irreversible coma or a permanently nonfunctioning brain. Both documents listed four criteria that signify that a person is no longer alive, even though such vital processes as breathing and blood circulation continue to be artificially maintained. These are: (1) lack of response to external stimuli; (2) no movement or breathing; (3) absence of reflexes, and (4) the confirmatory sign of a flat or isoelectric electroencephalogram (EEG). Therefore, the argument goes, death is a complex process. It consists in irreversible coma or a permanently nonfunctioning brain. A sign of this is a flat EEG. The absence of electrical activity in the brain is evidence that a person is dead, even though other vital processes may be mechanically continued. These vital processes may therefore be terminated for an organ or heart transplant. So, also, at the embryonic stage of life, a flat EEG should be accepted as a sign that an organism is not a living human person but only living tissue. Hence, for a good reason, these vital processes may be terminated.

This argument has a number of obvious weaknesses. One is that the other signs of life, e.g., reflex movements, are present in the embryo. More important is the fact that it is not the comatose state itself but the irreversibility of the coma that is the decisive factor in determining death. The absence of electrical activity in the brain is not permanent or final in the embryo. Just the opposite is true: its potentialities for full human life and personhood set it apart as quite different from a being whose permanently nonfunctioning brain signals that he is dead.

Joseph Donceel, S. J., thinks that in discussing the question of the beginning of human life, we ought to take another look at the Aristotelian-Thomistic thesis of delayed animation or, as he prefers to call it, delayed hominization.[27] Thomas's teaching that the human soul is not created until some time has elapsed in the developmental process of the embryo, he argues, does not have its foundation in outdated biology but in sound philosophy. According to Thomistic hylomorphism, the soul is the substantial form of man. But matter cannot receive its specific form until it is proportioned to it; that is to say, the human body must reach a certain stage of development and complexification before it can receive a human form or soul. The spiritual or rational anima cannot exist except in a highly organized body.

Donceel argues that Thomistic hylomorphism, while probably not defined at the Council of Vienne, always has and still does occupy a favored position in the Catholic church. What is more, delayed hominization is more in accord with modern philosophy's antidualistic explanation of man as embodied spirit, as the body of his soul as well as the soul of his body. Donceel concludes: "I feel certain that there is no human person until several weeks [of gestation] have elapsed."

Donceel's arguments have gained the interest and support of other Catholic theologians. Robert Springer, S. J., gives this verdict: "Donceel has uncovered strong historical evidence for his thesis, precedent in official teaching, and theological support to be reckoned with. Join to these his point of the kinship of hylomorphism with modern philosophy and his interpretation of the latest biological findings. It all adds up to a respectable case for delayed hominization. Taking a transtemporal view, we may conclude that the Catholic community enfolds a philosophico-theological pluralism on the question of immediate hominization."[28]

A fair conclusion about the beginning of human life has been expressed by Bernard Häring: "At this present stage of fetology, we cannot state a specific or accurate moment of hominization, although there is never any doubt of the developing process. As the fetus develops, there is an increasing degree of certainty that it has become a human being. On the other hand, there is also a growing consensus that not before implantation, and perhaps not even before the development of the basic brain structure, is individualization a full reality. Therefore, at this stage, there is a higher probability that we are not yet faced with a full human being."[29]

The best answer, therefore, to the question of when human life begins is that one cannot be absolutely sure. The fetus is certainly more than prehuman organic matter. Human life exists at least potentially from the moment of conception. And it is quite likely that it exists from the beginning in the sense of being matter which is activated by a human soul. But there is no way that one can be certain from the evidence available. This, I think, is the only honest conclusion one can draw from the empirical and philosophical data.

Contemporary Theological Opinion

The fundamental premise behind the common Catholic teaching on abortion is that the child in the womb has the same right to life as any other innocent human person. In a public address delivered on 26 November 1951, Pope Pius XII said: "Innocent human life, in whatsoever condition it is found, is withdrawn, from the very first moment of its existence, from any direct deliberate attack. This is a fundamental right of the human person, which is of general value in the Christian conception of life; hence as valid for the life still hidden within the womb of the mother as for the life already born and developing outside of her; as much opposed to direct abortion as to the direct killing of the child before, during or after its birth. Whatever foundation there may be for the distinction between these various phases of the development of life that is born or still unborn, in profane and ecclesiastical law, all these cases involve a grave and unlawful attack upon the inviolability of human life."[30]

A few weeks earlier (29 October 1951) he had said: "Now the infant is 'man' even though it be not yet born, to the same degree and through the same title as the mother."[31]

Once it is established as a premise that the life of the unborn child has the same inviolability as that of any innocent person, the conclusions come easily. The fetus may not be killed directly, but only indirectly and for a proportionate reason. Among Catholic theologians there have been some disputes about the application of the principle of double effect to particular cases. They have generally allowed one to remove a pregnant uterus for a proportionate reason, to use other surgical or chemical means to protect the mother even though an abortion may result, and to remove the fetal sac containing a live fetus (but not shell out the fetus) in an ectopic pregnancy. But until very recently they have all agreed that one may never directly destroy or abort a fetus for any reason.

Recently, however, there has been some discontent with this doctrine among Catholic theologians. Bernard Häring has suggested some refinements of Catholic teaching. His opinion is tentative, and he does not recommend its use in practice, since, he says, the presumption is in favor of the official magisterium and a doubt expressed by a theologian does not invalidate the official position. He then suggests two revisions. One concerns the case of therapeutic abortion. He relates the following case reported by a gynecologist: "I was once called upon to perform an operation on a woman in the fourth month of pregnancy, to remove a malign uterine tumor. On the womb there were numerous very thin and fragile varicose veins which bled profusely, and attempts to suture them only aggravated the bleeding. Therefore, in order to save the woman from bleeding to death, I opened the womb and removed the fetus. Thereupon the uterus contracted, the bleeding ceased, and the woman's life was saved. I was proud of what I had achieved, since the uterus of this woman, who was still childless, was undamaged and she could bear other children. But I had to find out later from a noted moralist that although I had indeed acted in good faith, what I had done was, in his eyes, *objectively* wrong. I would have been allowed to remove the bleeding uterus with the fetus itself, he said, but was not permitted to interrupt the pregnancy while leaving the womb intact. This latter, he said, constituted an immoral termination of pregnancy, though done for the purpose of saving the mother, while the other way would have been a lawful direct intention and action to save life. For him preservation of the woman's fertility and thereby, under some circumstances, preservation of the marriage itself, played no decisive role."[32]

Häring argues that the gynecologist acted correctly. The malice of abortion, he says, consists in an attack on the right of the fetus to live. The gynecologist in question did not deprive the fetus of its right to live, because it would not have survived even if he had not terminated the pregnancy. What he did was to serve life as best he could in the situation: he saved the mother's life and preserved her fertility. For Häring, abortion in the moral sense means more than the physical interruption of a pregnancy. It implies that one deprives the fetus of its right to live. But if the fetus has no chance to survive, the fact that the physician causes its biological death a bit early in order to save the mother does no harm to the right of the fetus, since it is not deprived of any personal activity.

Häring's second suggested revision is even more tentative. He simply raises the question about aborting a totally deformed fetus in which there is no development of the central nervous system and brain. He asks if it would be abortion in the moral sense to abort human biological life if there could never be any expression of humanity in it.

Robert Springer, S. J., also has expressed his dissatisfaction with an absolute prohibition of abortion: "The prohibition of direct abortion is an excellent rule, though not unexceptional. He who would attack innocent life must clearly establish his right to do so. The basic question, then, is not: Is it direct or indirect abortion? Rather it is: How great a value must be present to countervail the sacrifice of life?"[33]

Charles Curran takes the same view. In conflict situations where the mother's physical or mental health is endangered by a fetus that will not be able to survive, he suggests that the correct decision cannot be arrived at by considering only the physical act of abortion and its direct and indirect effects. Rather, he suggests, a better solution can be achieved by weighing the values at stake.[34] Specifically, Curran argues that individual human life does not begin until after the possibility of twinning and recombination has passed. After this point an abortion is permissible only if it is necessary "to save the life of the mother or to avert very grave psychological or physical harm to the mother with the realization that this must truly be grave harm that will perdure over some time and not just a temporary depression."[35]

After a long review of the contemporary literature on abortion, Richard McCormick expresses his own thinking on the matter. "Human life, as a basic good and the foundation for the enjoyment of other goods and rights, should be taken only when doing so is the lesser of two evils, all things considered. . . . 'Human life' refers to individual life from conception, or at least from 'the time at or after which it is settled whether there will be one or two or more distinct human individuals' (Ramsey). As this qualifier receives the continued discussion by theologians that it deserves, the benefit of the doubt should ordinarily be given to the fetus. To qualify as the lesser of two evils there is required, among other things, that there be at stake a human life or its moral equivalent. 'Moral equivalent' refers to a good or value that is, in Christian assessment, comparable to life itself. . . . This is the *substance* of the Christian tradition if our best casuistry in other areas (e.g., just warfare) is carefully weighed and sifted; for the permissible exceptions with regard to life-taking (self-defense, just war, capital punishment, indirect killing) are all formulations and concretizations of what is viewed in the situation as the lesser human evil."[36] I believe that McCormick is right in saying that "this position represents an achievement which, in terms of existing evidence, it would be unscientific to deny and uncivilized to abandon."[37]

In summary, therefore, we should say that although the majority of Catholic theologians still support the teaching of the magisterium, which absolutely proscribes all direct abortion no matter what the reason, there is a sizable and growing number of contemporary Catholic theologians who are arguing that there are some exceptions to this general rule.

Although some theologians argue that it is right for the state in a pluralistic society to legalize or decriminalize abortion, no one is supporting abortion for convenience as a moral position. No one is suggesting that abortion is no more than another form of contraception or that the fetus is just tissue in the womb of the mother, merely a part of her body which may be removed for any reason at all.

Contemporary theologians are only returning to an earlier theological position, saying that the prohibition of abortion is not an absolute one. Ordinarily the purposeful destruction of a fetus is morally wrong. But exceptions to this rule have to be made when a proportionate value, another life or its moral equivalent, is at stake.

Assisting at Abortions

The legalizing of abortion has given rise to a new problem of conscience for some Catholic nurses, interns, and paramedical personnel working in public and non-Catholic health facilities. Should they cooperate in any way with the abortions that now are being performed in the hospitals and clinics in which they are working?

Those in charge of these health facilities are rightly concerned that every abortion be performed with maximum medical safety for the pregnant woman. Therefore, after the abortion they generally require the woman to stay for a time in a recovery room, where she will be kept under observation for possible postoperative complications such as abscess, hemorrhage, and so on. Such complications are unusual, but if they do develop they can present a severe threat to the woman's life, and in that event, immediate attention by trained personnel is critically important.

Preoperative care is also important. Before the abortion an intern interviews and examines the woman to learn about any other diseases she may have, to check her blood pressure, heart, lungs, and so forth, so that if any complications occur after the operation an accurate diagnosis can be promptly made. A surgical nurse is even more directly involved. Her job may be to set out the instruments, hand them to the doctor, and so on.

In some rare instances administrative policy has required interns, nurses, and paramedics to perform these services —if they refused, they were fired or asked to resign. But even in the past such cases were unusual. At the present time hospital personnel are generally given a free choice. If they ask to be excused from this work for reasons of conscience, the administration will honor their request and there will be no recrimination. In some places discriminatory hiring practices have shown up, and sometimes the official administrative policy is compromised by subtle pressures or punishment by the particular individuals in charge. But in most cases the official policy is carried out in practice as meticulously and fairly as possible.

This is the context in which the moral question arises. What is the moral responsibility of those who believe that abortion is immoral? Should they participate in any way, or should they ask to be excused for reasons of conscience?

In themselves preoperative and postoperative care are morally good. It is the abortion that is immoral, not the medical care for the health and safety of the woman. This is exactly the same kind of care that an intern or nurse would give at a perfectly moral operation. The problem is that here it is not given at a perfectly moral operation. It is given in connection with an abortion.

If it is given with internal approval of the abortion, it is what theologians call formal cooperation, which is never permissible precisely because of one's internal approval of an immoral act. The formal cooperator is an accomplice who personally intends and wills not only the preoperative and postoperative care but the abortion as well. He shares in the blame for the abortion because of his bad will.

But it is quite possible for someone to give preoperative and postoperative care without approving of the abortion. Such care given without internal approval of the abortion is not formal cooperation. Rather it is called material cooperation. Material cooperation is permissible only if one manifests his disapproval so as to prevent scandal and at the same time has a proportionately serious reason for cooperating.

Therefore, the difficult decision of conscience revolves around this question: Do I have a proportionately serious reason for materially cooperating in an abortion? It is obvious at once that no universal answer can be given. The correct decision will depend on a complex of competing values in the particular situation. However, some broad statements can be made to illustrate how Catholic moral theologians generally evaluate the issue.

Practically all theologians agree that material cooperation in an abortion would be justified if the intern or nurse were threatened with some serious harm, for example, losing one's position with considerable personal loss. Also, many theologians argue that even if Catholic interns or nurses could get equally good or even better positions elsewhere, it does not follow necessarily that they should resign their positions at state institutions, since the spiritual and moral good they can do there may easily compensate for their occasional material assistance at an abortion.

In the present situation, however, loss of job is seldom, if ever, an issue. Generally speaking, no one's job is on the line. In most health facilities individual decisions of conscience will be respected without recrimination. And, normally, no serious harm will be caused to anyone if Catholic nurses and interns ask to be excused from assisting at abortions. What this means is that, ordinarily, there will be no proportionate reason to justify their material cooperation in abortions.

Therefore, as a normal rule in the present circumstance, Catholic nurses, interns, and paramedics should ask to be excused for reasons of personal conscience from assisting at abortions in any way. Preoperative and postoperative care can easily be given by others who have no conscientious objections to abortion.

This rule, of course, is not absolute. Certainly there will be exceptions to it. Emergency situations may develop in which a Catholic would be morally obliged to give postoperative care to a woman in need of it. And there may be other considerations of good to be accomplished or harm to be avoided which in a particular situation would justify material assistance.

But in the absence of such serious reasons, a Catholic

should abstain from any assistance directly connected with abortions. Although abortion is no longer a crime, it is still a sin. It is not enough for a Catholic merely to believe this internally. He should give visible witness to his convictions.

Hopefully, this common witness will say something to the medical profession and perhaps help sensitize others to the value of human life, whereas failure to give practical testimony could be scandalous in that it would tend to confirm the convictions of those who place less value on the lives of unborn children.[38]

CHAPTER 8

EUTHANASIA

Dr. John Farrell, professor of surgery at the University of Miami School of Medicine, once told a chapter of the American Council of Surgeons: "I submit that the deathbed scenes I witness are not particularly dignified. The family is shoved out into the corridor by the physical presence of intravenous stands, suction machines, oxygen tanks and tubes emanating from every natural and several surgically induced orifices. The last words, if the patient has not been comatose for the past forty-eight hours, are lost behind an oxygen mask. I discuss this, not because I have an answer to the problem but because it is a very real problem which all of us must face."[1]

In an address delivered at the Consultation on Medicine and Theology on 7 April 1967, Dr. Edward Rynearson, emeritus consultant in internal medicine at the Mayo Clinic, told the doctors that they should not be keeping dead people alive. He related the case of a woman in a Rochester nursing home who had been kept alive artificially for five years in a comatose state at a cost of $50,000. When she died an autopsy revealed that she "had no brain."[2]

In our Western culture in general and among members of the medical profession in particular there is not much sympathy for euthanasia. All the efforts of medical science are turned in the opposite direction, toward the preservation of human life for as long as possible. The Hippocratic oath taken by physicians contains the promise to refuse to give a "deadly drug to any, though it be asked of me." When originally composed, this vow probably was meant merely to exclude physicians from becoming accessories to familial murders and political assassinations by poison. Today its meaning has been broadened to include the repudiation of euthanasia.

Margaret Mead has suggested that the recent fuss and squeamishness about heart transplants reflects nothing more than our contemporary reluctance to terminate human life. Three arguments are customarily raised against heart transplants, she says, but the first two are merely evasions of the real question that men have on their minds. The first is the argument that if two people need a heart and we only have one, who is going to decide who gets it? This argument, of course, has nothing to do with hearts. It can be asked equally about food, antibiotics, vaccines, or any other medical or surgical aid. We have a shortage of nearly everything in the world. This means that we go out and try to produce more, not that we withhold what we have from everybody on the grounds of fairness. The second argument also avoids the real issue. It claims that heart transplants are too experimental, too hazardous to be undertaken with a human being. But when a patient's life already is at stake, it is certainly reasonable for him to take a risk—he has so much to gain and so little to lose. As Margaret Mead says: "The real issue that we are talking about—and attempting to dodge by bringing in these other questions—is the issue of whether the physician should ever be asked to perform, on a patient who still has any life left in him at all, an operation which means certain death."[3]

Our contemporary reluctance to enter into the business

of terminating human lives is shaped by two factors. One is the undeniable increase in modern times in moral sensitivity to the value of human life and to the inviolability of the unique human person. It is an appropriation by our modern culture, for a variety of reasons, of values that are at the heart of the message of Jesus.

The other factor is our lingering shock and revulsion at what occurred in relatively recent Western history in Nazi Germany. The "Law for the Prevention of Hereditarily Diseased Posterity," promulgated in July 1933, and Hitler's euthanasia decree, signed on 1 September 1939, led to the "merciful" gassing of mentally afflicted adults and deformed and idiotic children as well as to the systematic attempt to exterminate certain races, primarily the Jews, declared to be inferior. It has been estimated that at least 275,000 people perished in the German euthanasia centers. The number may have been substantially higher. Obviously, the humane termination of the life of a person who is painfully and incurably ill and who asks for a painless release from the excruciating process of dying is quite different from compulsory euthanasia or genocide. Even so, the horror produced by Dachau and Buchenwald has caused contemporary men to distrust the idea of granting anyone the right and power to decide who shall live and who shall die.

Theological Opinion

What was going on in the German euthanasia centers during the 1930s and early 1940s no doubt was known to Dietrich Bonhoeffer and perhaps influenced the strong stand he took against euthanasia. All deliberate killing of innocent life, Bonhoeffer says, is arbitrary. He reduces all the arguments for euthanasia to two—consideration for the sick and consideration for the healthy—and he says that neither argument is convincing. If one is truly concerned about the sick person, one will not kill him without his consent, and the sick person may not give consent without incurring the guilt of suicide, which is at bottom a sin of lack of faith. God alone has the right to put an end to life because he gave it and because he alone knows the destiny he has appointed for it. Nor can we terminate human life out of concern for the healthy, because life has an inherent God-given value that transcends its utility. Not only is it socially dangerous for men to begin to make utilitarian discriminations about whose life is worth living; in the sight of God there is no life that is not worth living.

Bonhoeffer does suggest two possible exceptions to his otherwise uncompromising stand against euthanasia. One is the borderline case of people who have contracted plague on a ship where there is no possibility of isolating the sick from the healthy, so that only through the death of the sick can the others be saved. The other possible exception is the case in which a doctor does not do everything possible to prevent a man from dying. "There is a difference," Bonhoeffer says, "between allowing to die and killing. It is in any case not always possible in life to give effect to all conceivable means for the postponement of death, and yet this is still fundamentally different from intentional killing." But in principle the Bible sums up his judgment in a sentence in Exodus 23:7: "The innocent thou shalt not slay."[4]

Karl Barth is even more strongly opposed to euthanasia: "It is for God and God alone to make an end of human life." He admits no possibility of any *ultima ratio* that might signal an exception. Euthanasia is murder, the usurpation of the sovereign right of God over life and death. There is no possibility of any clear command of God to do otherwise in an exceptional case. Euthanasia is never justified, he says, "even when it is not so much a matter of active killing as of the passive failure to apply the stimulants . . . which artificially prolong life." However, at the very end of his consideration of euthanasia, he cautiously raises the question of the possibility of fanaticism and foolishness and even human arrogance in prolonging life painfully and artificially with every possible means to the last possible moment. He says that this may raise an exceptional case, but that we will have to await further developments before we can reach a clear judgment.[5]

Paul Ramsey, on the other hand, seizes on the distinction between killing and allowing to die. Christians have wisely seen a difference, he says, between ordinary and extraordinary means of preserving life and beneath this distinction have recognized a difference between prolonging life and prolonging dying, which is tantamount to forbidden and useless torture. Which means are to be counted as ordinary and which extraordinary cannot be determined concretely outside of circumstances. The categories are relative and changing. A major surgical operation would some years ago have been extraordinary means; today it would be considered quite ordinary in most cases.

It is certainly required, Ramsey says, "even in grievous illness that every effort be made to save life." But when a particular patient's dying has taken "irreversible control" it is another matter. "Have we not gone too far," he asks, "in thoughtlessly supposing that any means for prolonging life, once it is made available, becomes ordinary and morally mandatory upon both patient and doctor?" Ramsey does not do the appropriate line-drawing himself, but suggests that moralists and doctors work together "to enlarge again the categories of extraordinary means which are morally dispensible, and to explore the difference between saving life and prolonging dying." Assistance of life should not become useless torture and respect for life should include respect for the dignity of the dying man."[6]

Catholic moralists have shown considerably more tolerance than Protestants toward discontinuing or not using certain means to preserve life. They are agreed that a man must use ordinary means to preserve his life, and they define *ordinary means* as "not only normal food, drink and rest but all medicines, treatments, and operations which offer a reasonable hope of benefit and which can be obtained and used without excessive expense, pain or other inconvenience."[7]

They also are agreed that a man may use extraordinary means, but that, generally speaking, he is not obliged to do so. He would be obliged to use extraordinary means only if the success of these means were very likely and the patient's life were necessary to his dependents, the common good, or his own spiritual welfare. *Extraordinary means* is defined as "all medicines, treatments, and operations which cannot be obtained or used without excessive expense, pain or other inconvenience for the patient or others, or which if used would not offer a reasonable hope of benefit to the patient."[8] Accordingly, means to preserve life are considered extraordinary if, here and now, they are very costly, very unusual, very painful, very difficult, or very dangerous, or if the inconvenience of using them is not proportionate to the good effects that can be expected from them.

There is a significant difference, therefore, between the meaning assigned the terms *ordinary* and *extraordinary* by physicians and the meaning intended by Catholic moralists. The physician usually considers ordinary whatever means are standard, orthodox, or established medicines or procedures within the limits of availability; he considers extraordinary a medicament or procedure that is fanciful, bizarre, experimental, incompletely established, unorthodox, or not recognized.[9] For the Catholic moralist, on the other hand, the ordinariness of the means is measured by two factors—convenience and utility.

Catholic theologians have not shared Ramsey's reluctance to engage in specific line-drawing. Their detailed casuistry does not provide ready-made decisions for particular situations. It does show in clear and concrete terms the direction of their thinking. It would be instructive to take a look at some of this casuistry in order to appreciate how far Catholic moralists are willing to go in this area in contrast to the hesitant approach of Bonhoeffer, Barth, and even Ramsey.

Ramsey is concerned only with the case of the person who is dying—not, of course, in the sense that all of us are dying, nor merely in the sense that one's life is threatened by a curable illness. He is concerned with the terminal case, in which a patient's dying has taken "irreversible control." In grievous illness, he says, it is certainly required that every effort be made to save life. Catholic moralists, however, say plainly that even a man whose illness is not terminal, even a man who has a medically curable disease, is not obliged to use extraordinary means to effect a cure.

Some concrete examples reveal how liberal the majority of Catholic moralists are in this area. Any financial expense, for instance, that would be a grave burden for an individual is considered extraordinary means. Making his judgment in terms of the value of money in 1956, Edwin Healy, S.J., held that no one, no matter how wealthy he may be, is bound to spend more than two thousand dollars to preserve his life.[10] Six months in bed or in an iron lung is also extraordinary means, and so is a surgical operation that would be very painful, provoke very great fear or horror in a patient, or involve very serious danger of death. The danger of death is considered very serious if the mortality rate of the particular operation is over 10 percent; such special circumstances as old age or a weak heart may make any operation an extraordinary means.

Healy, Kelly, Ford, McFadden, and other Catholic moralists were making judgments like these during the 1950s and 1960s, and they were talking about the means that must be used for those with curable diseases. In discussing the means required for the dying, i.e., those terminal patients whose dying has taken irreversible control, they were even more lenient. They generally held that such artificial means as intravenous feeding, oxygen, blood transfusions, or chemical stimulants are extraordinary means because they are actually useless in the effort to save life and do not offer reasonable hope of any notable benefit to the patient. Therefore, the dying are generally obliged to use only such natural means as food and drink to stay alive.

Gerald Kelly, S.J., has written: "I am often asked whether such things as oxygen and intravenous feeding must be used to prolong the life of a patient, already well prepared for death, and now in a terminal coma. In my opinion, the circumstances of this case make it obvious that the non-use of artificial life-sustainers is not the same as mercy-killing; and I see no reason why even the most delicate professional standard should call for their use. In fact, it seems to me that, apart from very special circumstances, the artificial means not only need not but should not be used, once the coma is reasonably diagnosed as terminal. Their use creates expense and nervous strain without conferring any real benefit."[11]

A similar case is that of a cancer patient who is conscious, has developed a tolerance to painkilling drugs so that they give only brief relief, and will live for several more weeks unless the doctor pulls the plug on the artificial respirator and removes the tubes for intravenous feeding. Some Catholic moralists like Joseph Sullivan allow the discontinuance of these artificial aids since they are not useful means to save life.[12] Kelly agrees in principle but expresses fear of misunderstanding and scandal: "I fear that the abrupt ceasing to nourish a conscious patient might appear to be a sort of 'Catholic euthanasia' to many who cannot appreciate the fine distinction between omitting an *ordinary* means and omitting a *useless* ordinary means."[13]

Closely allied to this question is another: If a patient

has two fatal diseases, one curable and the other not, should the physician continue to treat the curable disease? For instance, should a physician always treat and cure pneumonia in an aged and senile patient? Or should a physician prescribe insulin for a terminal cancer patient who develops diabetes? Or must a diabetic patient who develops terminal cancer continue his insulin injections?

The physician as a scientist is inclined to see his task as treating and curing diseases. The moralist, who is not a scientist, gives the physician a somewhat different job description. The physician's mission is to cure people and save their lives. His job is patient-centered, not disease-centered. As Paul Ramsey once observed, "Doctors do not treat diseases, though they often conquer them. They treat patients, and here finally all fail."[14]

This subtle nuance in perspective makes a great practical difference. In the case of the patient who has two fatal diseases, one that can be checked and another that is terminal—for instance, a terminal cancer patient who developes diabetes or a diabetic patient who develops an incurable cancer, or a slowly deteriorating senile old man who develops pneumonia—the ethical conclusion is that the disease which may be cured or checked need not be treated. The reason is simply that the treatment in such circumstances is not a useful remedy. The treatment will halt one of the diseases, but it will not confer significant benefit on the patient. The subject of medical treatment is the patient who has two diseases. It is not the individual diseases one by one; only a narrowly scientific view would say it is.

In deciding whether one is obliged to use insulin for diabetes or antibiotics for pneumonia in such cases, one cannot merely ask whether the treatment will cure or check the disease. One must ask whether the treatment will be useful and beneficial for the patient, whose dying has already taken irreversible control. One does not realistically prescind from an advanced and terminal cancer in answering that question.

It is, of course, first of all the right of the patient himself, not the doctor, to decide whether extraordinary measures should be initiated or discontinued. If the patient is conscious and rational, that is, able to understand and evaluate the situation, it is up to him to decide the issue, and the doctor should respect his wishes.

But if the patient is unconscious or unable to decide rationally, theoretically his nearest kin should make the decision for him. Practically, however, the relatives are often the worst judges of what should be done when someone they love is dying. The members of the immediate family often feel enormous guilt, not because of what they have done in the past, but because of what they imagine they should or might have done to show the love they now so keenly feel. As a result, they want everything possible done for the patient now. They want to prolong his living to the last possible moment and beyond any reasonable moral warrant. They cannot bear the added guilt that would come from a decision to discontinue any means that might delay the death of the one they love.

In such a situation it can easily become the responsibility of the doctor to take the lead in suggesting what should and what should not be done, what in his judgment would be best for the dying man. In this way he can help the family come to the right decision and reduce considerably the burden of a decision which otherwise they could not bear. Also there will be situations in which the family cannot or should not be consulted. Then the doctor will have to make the decision himself according to what he judges to be the best interest of the patient.

Pope Pius XII taught that a man has the right to die in dignity. He affirmed in principle the approach of the Catholic moralists, without endorsing all of their casuistic judgments, in an address on 24 November 1957: "Natural reason and Christian morals say that man (and whoever is entrusted with the task of taking care of his fellowman) has the right and duty in case of serious illness to take the necessary treatment for the preservation of life and health. This duty that one has toward himself, toward God, toward the human community, and in most cases toward certain determined persons, derives from well-ordered charity, from submission to the Creator, from social justice, as well as from devotion toward one's family. But normally one is held to use only ordinary means—according to circumstances of persons, places, times, and cultures—that is to say, means that do not involve any grave burden for oneself or another. A more strict obligation would be too burdensome for most men and would render the attainment of the higher, more important good too difficult. Life, health, all temporal activities are in fact subordinated to spiritual ends. On the other hand, one is not forbidden to take more than strictly necessary steps to preserve life and health, as long as he does not fail in some more serious duty."[15]

Accordingly, the pope said, if the medical or surgical means have little hope of success and are "such a burden for the family that one cannot in all conscience impose it upon them, they can lawfully insist that the doctor should discontinue these attempts."[16]

Admittedly, some of the specific casuistry that has been done by Catholic moralists in this area has been extreme and is indefensible. But in general it reveals a more reasonable and practical attitude toward life and death than the more squeamish and hesitant positions of such Protestant ethicists as Bonhoeffer, Barth, and even Ramsey. It does not reflect any fundamental depreciation of the value of human life; rather, it formulates some common-sense perceptions. Biological life is a limited, relative value which we do not need to protect at all costs. There are limits to men's endurance and to the burdens that they can bear even in the effort to continue to live. What is more, in the protection of life we are not obliged to do what is practically useless or what offers little hope of significant benefit. And finally, as Ramsey points out, "to die is one way of being a human creature and to be allowed to die a precious human right."

Euthanasia By Direct Killing

Up to this point our analysis has presumed that there is a significant moral difference between direct killing and allowing to die. It will be useful to examine this assumption and to inquire whether the direct killing of sick, crippled, or dying people might also sometimes be permissible.

The killing of sick people is not and probably never has been an extremely popular cause. Richard Cabot once described euthanasia as "that ancient and reliable novelty . . . which newspapers trick out afresh each year in August when politics are dull and there is a dearth of copy." But there is and has been some support for it from such able and conscientious men as Plato, Seneca, and Joseph Fletcher. That there is something important to be said for their position is reflected in the fact that although euthanasia is allowed nowhere in the United States, anyone who is convicted of mercy killing usually is given a mild sentence or is set free without any penalty at all.

G. K. Chesterton once remarked that while the proponents of euthanasia begin by seeking only the deaths of those who are a nuisance to themselves, they will soon broaden their objective to include those who are a nuisance to others. But it is not easy to prove any necessary connection between voluntary and involuntary euthanasia, and it is not fair to assume one. Voluntary euthanasia is one thing; compulsory euthanasia is quite another. It will be useful to keep the two separate in our discussion.

A strong case for euthanasia without the consent of the

individual who is being put to death has been made by Joseph Fletcher. Writing in *The Atlantic* in 1968, he limits his recommendation to certain classes of mentally retarded children. He does not insist that euthanasia is always the right thing to do in all cases of retardation. Such an insistence would be another absurd legalism—after all, idiots, cretins, and morons are not the same.

Fletcher is particularly concerned about the embryonic anomaly called Down's syndrome, popularly known as mongolism. In a manner consistent with his utilitarian ethic he argues that the principle that the end does not justify the means is an old and irrational bromide. The only ethical question worth asking is, "Is the flame worth the candle?" Life is not always good. When it is not good it deserves neither protection nor preservation. In the case of Down's syndrome, he argues, it is obvious that the end everybody wants is death. Therefore, it would be straightforward and honest to mercifully kill the infant, since the mongoloid's life is not worth living and imposes a great burden on others. In fact, he says, the mongoloid child is not a human person, for to be human is to be self-aware, rational, and interpersonally related to others.

Our reluctance to extinguish mercifully the lives of such anomalies as mongoloids, instead of keeping them biologically alive until they die of natural causes, is the result, he says, of superstitious religious taboos or of a selfish, fearful, and idolatrous vitalism which claims that "all life is sacred and my life most of all." It is inhuman, archaic, and irresponsible to pretend that only God can make an end to life. The real guilt is in not saving the money that is wasted in keeping a monstrosity alive and using it to raise a living and learning child.[17]

It is not easy to accommodate an ethic of compulsory euthanasia within the spirit of the Christian Gospel. Nor is it easy to dismiss a deformed or retarded child as not a human person. Such a child is more accurately described as a seriously crippled human being who is incurable at the present stage of development of medical science.

For a Christian the value of a human being is more than can be calculated in utilitarian terms. He is not subordinated to the interests of other men or the State. The Christian tradition is reflected in the words of Pope Pius XII: "The Apostle with good reason admonishes us: 'Much more those that seem to be the more feeble members of the Body, are more necessary, and such as we think to be the less honorable members of the Body, about these we put more abundant honor.' Conscious of the obligations of our high office, We deem it necessary to reiterate this grave statement today, when to Our profound grief We see the bodily-deformed, the insane and those suffering from hereditary disease at times deprived of their lives, as though they were a useless burden to society. And this procedure is hailed by some as a new discovery of human progress, and as something that is altogether justified by the common good. Yet what sane man does not recognize that this not only violates the natural and divine law written in the heart of every man, but flies in the face of every sensibility of civilized humanity? The blood of these victims, all the dearer to our Redeemer because deserving of greater pity, 'cried to God from the earth.' "[18]

Writing fourteen years earlier, Fletcher had limited his proposal to voluntary euthanasia, euthanasia performed only with the consent of the patient.[19] The model legislation he would like to see enacted is incorporated in a bill once proposed in the state of New York by the Euthanasia Society of America. Essentially its provisions are as follows:

1. Any sane person over twenty-one years old, suffering from an incurably painful and fatal disease, may petition a court of record for euthanasia, in a signed and attested

document, with an affidavit from the attending physician that in his opinion the disease is incurable.
2. The court shall appoint a commission of three, of whom at least two shall be physicians, to investigate all aspects of the case and to report back to the court whether the patient understands the purpose of his petition and comes under the provisions of the act.
3. Upon a favorable report by the commission the court shall grant the petition, and *if it is still wanted by the patient* euthanasia may be administered by a physician or any other person chosen by the patient or by the commission.[20]

The crucial element in voluntary euthanasia is that the individual freely decides that he wants to be put to death. No one else can make the decision for him. There are, of course, a host of dangers here. The most serious is that a man's consent to euthanasia may be only apparently free. He may not be able psychologically to make a fully free and human choice because of his physical or mental condition. Or his consent might be manipulated or engineered subtly or not so subtly by pressures brought to bear on him by others who also have an interest at stake. Or societal expectations could become such that an individual would be afraid or ashamed to ask others to bear the burden of keeping him alive, so that in certain circumstances he would see no other practical option than to sign up for euthanasia. These risks probably never can be totally eliminated. Still, it is possible for a person to make a fully free and human choice of death, and it is this case that we must consider.

Fletcher rightly points out that the question we are now talking about is the morality of suicide: Does a man ever have the right to directly kill himself? The issue, Fletcher says, is not one of life or death. The issue is what kind of death, a peaceful or an agonized one. He argues that man need not leave this decision to chance or fate or the will of God. He should make a rational decision, and it would be reasonable for him to prefer a painless release from a useless and excruciating process of physical and personal disintegration.

To clinch his argument Fletcher cites the great wisdom shown in the decision of Charlotte Perkins Gilman, who chose self-euthanasia rather than a degenerative death by cancer. Her final words, typed by her own hand, were: "A last duty. Human life consists in mutual service. No grief, no pain, misfortune or 'broken heart' is excuse for cutting off one's life while any power of service remains. But when all usefulness is over, when one is assured of an imminent and unavoidable death, it is the simplest of human rights to choose a quick and easy death in place of a slow and horrible one. Public opinion is changing on this subject. The time is approaching when we shall consider it abhorrent to our civilization to allow a human being to lie in prolonged agony which we should mercifully end in any other creature. Believing this choice to be of social service in promoting wider views on this question, I have preferred chloroform to cancer."[21]

Christians of course understand that suffering and pain are physical evils. It is not without precedent for a man faced with a miserable death to wish that cup to pass from him. But it is the New Testament, not some perverse masochism, that invites us to see a transcendent meaning and redemptive purpose in physical suffering. This does not mean that the Christian does not recognize physical suffering as evil, does nothing to relieve it, or chases after it with the fanaticism of some of his religious ascendants. It does mean that he does not interpret the inevitable presence of suffering and death in God's creation as empty of all possible purpose and meaning as long as he continues to believe in the meaning of the cross and his union with the Crucified.

The ethical question is not solved simply by restricting

euthanasia to the voluntary sort. The ethical question is not "What does a man want?" The question is "What ought he to want?" Utility is not the only measure that one should use in trying to answer this question.

A Needed Clarification

There is a growing medical, legal, and theological consensus that one need not, in fact ought not to, use extraordinary means to prolong the lives of patients who are terminally ill. Prolonging the process of dying through artificial means provides no important benefit and is generally useless and unreasonable. There is, in other words, a human right to die.

There is not the same support for directly interfering in order to hasten death. The general reluctance to directly or actively cause death appears to reflect a common-sense perception that there is a significant moral difference between killing and allowing to die. Fletcher has put the question clearly. He says that this distinction is dishonest, that it merely signals an unwillingness to make and implement a responsible human decision in an active way.

One must admit that there is no perfect clarity here. One has to wonder whether the distinction between an active and a passive response to dying is merely the consequence of a unilateral concern about the physical nature of the act of killing.

Bernard Häring's analysis of another case—that of a captured spy who kills himself under his government's orders to protect vitally secret information—may provide some illumination. Catholic theologians generally have judged that this direct act of killing is an illicit suicide even though done for a noble purpose. But Häring says that "it is conceivably a moot question whether taking one's life in these circumstances is suicide in the strict moral sense."[22] One might raise the same question about the direct administration of a lethal drug to a dying person (supposing his consent). Is this suicide in the strict moral sense? Is the physical act of deliberately taking one's life always and necessarily suicide in the moral sense?

Charles Curran has raised the same question: "At the particular time when death is fast approaching, the primary moral question does not seem to revolve explicitly around the notion of man's dominion over his life. The problem centers on the difference between not giving something or the withdrawal of something necessary for life and the positive giving of something to bring about death. Is the difference between the two types of action enough to warrant the total condemnation of positively interfering? I do not think so; Catholic theologians should explore the possibility of interfering to hasten the dying process."[23]

Obviously there is a lack of clarity here, and we should remain open to the possibility of a further revision of our ethical policy. But at present I do not think that we should abandon a moral distinction between active and passive euthanasia in terminal cases. Curran wisely cautions that in their deliberations theologians would have to consider the societal effects of abandoning this distinction in practice. Harmon Smith expresses the same reservation. He thinks that the active administration of death-inducing or life-terminating agents "is not needed if we properly understand the dispensability (i.e. the non-mandatoriness) of both extraordinary and ordinary means which are not remedies." The line, he admits, is a fine one but "is reinforced by the awareness that medical science and technology have developed many possibilities for which we have not yet developed the ethical wisdom and moral stamina necessary for exercising humanely responsible control."[24]

The point between passively withholding artificial means and actively giving lethal agents is a practical and reasonable place to draw a line. Crossing that line at this time would set human beings on a road whose direction is dangerous and whose end is obscure.[25]

Part Four

The Human Mind

CHAPTER 9

PSYCHOSURGERY AND BEHAVIOR CONTROL

In the summer of 1935, at the Second International Neurology Congress in London, Dr. Carlyle Jacobsen reported on the work being done by him and his colleague, Prof. John F. Fulton, in their Yale University laboratory, where they were engaged in the modification of the behavior of monkeys and chimpanzees by the surgical destruction of the prefrontal area of the cerebral cortex. After Jacobsen's presentation a Portuguese neuropsychiatrist, Dr. Egas Moniz, rose to ask why these same surgical procedures could not be used to relieve anxiety states in man.

Both Jacobsen and Fulton were shocked at the thought. Nonetheless, Egas Moniz persuaded Almeida Lima to perform under his supervision a prefrontal lobotomy on a human being. The first operation was performed in Lisbon on 12 November 1935 on a mental patient "who had proven refractory to other methods of treatment."

Twenty more operations followed, and the results were mixed. All of the patients survived: seven were considered recovered, and seven were said to have improved. In 1949 Moniz shared the Nobel Prize in Physiology and Medicine with Walter Hess "for his discovery of the therapeutic value of prefrontal leucotomy in certain psychoses."

In September 1936 Drs. Walter Freeman and James Watts of George Washington University in Washington, D.C., introduced Dr. Moniz's technique in the United States. Under their direction the operation was refined and perfected. It is estimated that since 1936 about forty thousand prefrontal lobotomies have been performed in the United States.

By the late 1950s there was a sharp decline in the practice of psychosurgery. A number of newly discovered psychoactive drugs had been proven useful in treating psychiatric disorders. Also there had been many reports of undesirable side effects of psychosurgery, such as personality deterioration, a lack of planning ability and foresight, a general blunting of emotional responsiveness, and so on.

Although there was a rapid decline in the amount of psychosurgery performed after the mid-1950s, research continued in an effort to help patients who were not responsive to psychoactive drugs or other therapeutic measures. Today newer and much more precise surgical techniques have been developed, and other portions of the brain, for instance, the amygdala and the hypothalamus, are ablated.

Dr. William Scoville, the president of the International Society of Psychiatric Surgery, reports that today about six hundred brain operations are performed each year in the United States for purely psychiatric disease, and more are performed to alleviate pain, epilepsy, movement disorders, and aggression.[1]

Because the subject of psychosurgery remains highly controversial, it is difficult to get an accurate and objective evaluation of the contemporary techniques. Perhaps the fairest evaluation is that given by Dr. Elliot Valenstein: "The problem of evaluation of the newer psychosurgical techniques remains difficult, since many of the shortcomings of the earlier lobotomy studies are still evident. It is also necessary to recognize that there has been a clear shift in the type of patients selected for psychosurgery. Originally, only chronic psychotic patients who were considered otherwise hopeless were picked for surgery. Gradually it became clear that the prognosis was very poor for such patients. Today the patients considered to be the best candidates are those with tensions, anxieties, phobias, depressions, obsessions, compulsions, and severe hypochondriacal symptoms. As a group the patients are not nearly as deteriorated as the earlier lobotomy patients, but this does not mean that their symptoms are mild. The patients may be constantly anxious or depressed and suicide attempts are not uncommon. In some, the phobias, obsessions, or physical complaints may completely block any kind of normal existence. . . . The evaluative studies of the newer psychosurgical procedures tend to have smaller numbers of subjects who have been followed for shorter periods of time. In general, insufficient details are provided, but the results reported are favorable in terms of psychiatric improvement, work adjustment, and low incidence of serious intellectual and personality changes or physical complications. It may be important to bear in mind, however, that these reports have customarily been presented by those doing the surgery—there has not been sufficient interest generated to sponsor a more impartial, as well as more thorough, evaluation."[2]

Science owes a great debt to Dr. José M. P. Delgado, who pioneered the development of many brain stimulation techniques. But his flamboyant and dramatic exhibitions have given rise to a greatly exaggerated notion in the popular mind about the power of modern brain controllers. To take only one example, Delgado once implanted a radio-controlled electrode in the brain of a brave bull, a species bred to aggressively charge any human being in his view. Dr. Delgado stood alone in the arena and faced the charging bull. When the charging bull was within a few feet of Delgado, the doctor calmly pressed a button on a transmitter in his hand, sending a signal to the brave bull's brain, and the bull abruptly stopped in his tracks, becoming, according to a report in the *New York Times*, "as gentle as Ferdinand."

This sensational experiment has been interpreted as proof that aggressive behavior can now be controlled by brain manipulation. The truth is considerably more complex than that. Delgado's electrode affected the caudate nucleus, which is one of several brain structures that plays an important role in controlling physical movement and fine muscular responses. A modern phrenology which asserted that there is a specific area of the brain controlling aggressiveness would be regarded with the greatest suspicion by most contemporary brain physiologists and neurologists. It is quite unlikely that the brain is organized into neat areas that match our labels for describing human emotions and behavior. As Dr. Valenstein says, "To conclude from [Delgado's] demonstration that we are close to being able to selectively reduce aggression in the normal human being without producing many other effects seems, to put it as diplomatically as possible, very questionable at best."[3]

It is, of course, now possible to modify or diminish human aggressiveness by brain surgery or brain stimulation. But this does not imply that there is one precisely aggressive faculty which can be located in the brain. Brain surgery which reduces aggressiveness has other consequences as well. Most psychosurgeons agree that the changes produced by brain surgery are frequently general and nonspecific, are influenced by the individual personality of the patient, and are never wholly predictable.

The assumption that psychosurgery is now or soon will be an exact science and technique of controlling the minds, emotions, and wills of men is gaining some currency in the popular mind. Newspaper articles, picture magazines, and current novels and movies like Anthony Burgess's *A Clockwork Orange* and Michael Crichton's *The Terminal Man* have spread a fear that we are in grave danger of becoming a society of robots controlled and manipulated by brain surgeons and brain stimulators. We are told that the new surgical and electronic techniques are now or soon will be perfected to such a point that they already represent a singularly potent and diabolical threat to human society and the human species. Think, we are told, of the power of a dictator who could electronically control the behavior of an entire population by means of electrodes implanted in their brains. Think of an omnipotent police state that could eliminate demonstrations, riots, revolutions, dissent, or any other form of "deviant" behavior. Think of a moralist who could make all men conform to a single code of ethics and uniform, approved patterns of thought and behavior, and be perfectly happy in their docile, obedient, and servile condition.

Dr. Steven Rose, head of the Brain Research Group at the Open University in England, gives a more realistic assessment of the situation. He says: "This threat is, I believe, still in the realm of science fiction. Granted that electrical control of mood *is* possible—and this does seem to be the case both in animals and humans—and also that radio-controlled implanted electrodes are already available—for such a technique to be applicable on any large scale would demand a degree of social acquiescence in being implanted which is hard to envisage, quite apart from demanding the production of doctors who would carry out the implantations and controllers who would presumably regulate a population's mood by the tuning of a radio dial. Traditional techniques of mass persuasion and mood change are likely to remain more practicable and more effective than this for the foreseeable future."[4] Common sense would suggest that any dictator who could persuade the population to submit to having parts of their brains excised or to having electrodes implanted in them would not need such fantastic tools; he would already have achieved his objective. As Dr. Vernon

H. Mark has said: "No drugs were needed to seduce the German population. The S.S. storm troopers did not have little electrodes implanted in their limbic systems. . . . My own claim is that the dangers of mass abuse are not sufficient to warrant preventing the very development of the techniques that might have very great therapeutic value for patients with organic brain disease."[5]

All this, of course, is not meant to imply that there are no dangers or moral problems involved in the manipulation of the human brain. It is only to say that we should not waste our time by mislocating them.

The Moral Concerns

In an address of 13 September 1952 Pope Pius XII said that a man may not submit to medical procedures which alleviate physical or psychic illness, but at the same time "involve the destruction or the diminution to a considerable and lasting extent of freedom—that is to say, of the human personality in its typical and characteristic functions. In that way man is degraded to the level of a purely sensory being—a being of acquired reflexes or a living automaton. Such a reversal of values is not permitted by the natural law."[6]

When this statement first appeared some doctors thought that the pope had condemned prefrontal lobotomies. But the Catholic moralists of the time assured them that he had not. The moralists' reading of the papal statement was that the pope was simply pointing out that in the proper hierarchy of values man's free personal life was the highest and should not be sacrificed for some lesser good. Psychosurgery, they judged, is to be morally evaluated according to the same canons as surgery in general and experimental surgery in particular. Specifically, this means that with the informed consent of the patient or his relatives, psychosurgery is justified in accord with the principle of totality.

Accordingly, the old *Ethical and Religious Directives for Catholic Hospitals* said: "Lobotomy is morally justifiable as a last resort in attempting to cure those who suffer from serious mental illness. It is not allowed when less extreme measures are reasonably available or in cases in which the probability of harm outweighs the probability of benefit."[7] Succinctly put, this means that psychosurgery is morally permitted when it is medically indicated. In other words, here good morality is simply good medical practice.

Today it is easier to make this same judgment about the morality of psychosurgery, since the modern techniques are more refined and the risk of deleterious effects has been reduced. Dr. William Scoville, president of the International Society of Psychiatric Surgery, expressed it this way: "The ethical question here is no different from the ethical problem in other surgical lesions of the body. Destructive surgery is done for cancer of vital organs and limbs, necessitating amputation and partial evisceration. The ethics of such surgery can best be simply stated: If surgery benefits overall function it is justified. If overall function is made worse by the operation than by the disease, then surgery is not justified. Certainly all surgical lesions of the brain are destructive of some function; but continuing mental disease may be more destructive of function. Surgical lesions can cut out pathological thought processes or 'sick circuits' so that there may result an impressive benefit in overall brain function, thus resulting in a happier and more productive social being."[8]

That, I believe, expresses the central principle that governs the morality of psychosurgery. But, unfortunately, the whole matter is not quite so simple. A good number of practical problems still remain to be settled. There are several important issues that keep coming up in the current discussion.

The first question concerns the appropriate subjects for psychosurgery. Should psychosurgery be used: (1) to improve all, even normal, human behavior, (2) to treat all abnormal behavior, or (3) to treat only abnormal behavior which is caused by an abnormality of the brain? What limits should we set to its use?

Practically no one advocates brain surgery as a means of improving all normal human behavior. The fact is that psychosurgery cannot achieve such a goal now and will not be able to in the foreseeable future. Besides, even if it were, the moral judgments that would have to be made about what counts as "improved behavior" would be very illusive. As Dr. Vernon Mark has pointed out, "moral values are social concerns, not medical ones in any presently recognized sense."[9]

Most of those writing on the topic argue that brain surgery should be performed only when a person's abnormal behavior can be traced to organic brain disease. Much violent behavior, for instance, is the product not of a diseased brain but of a diseased society. Moral, social, and political problems should not be treated by surgical means. They should be resolved by moral, social, and political means.

It is easy to accept this as a principle. But a problem often arises in neurological diagnosis. It is not always easy to tell in a specific case whether abnormal violence is due to brain dysfunction or to social or environmental causes. Dr. Vernon Mark relates the case of an airplane hijacker who recently killed one pilot and shot another: "Examination of this man afterward revealed he had been a neurological cripple for eleven years, ever since receiving a gunshot wound of the brain. Yet repeated tests, including hours of brainwave examinations, psychological testing and neurological assessment, failed to reveal the tremendous damage that had occurred in this man's emotional center or limbic brain."[10]

Similarly, George Gershwin, the composer, was treated psychiatrically for many years, while a tumor was growing in the limbic system of his brain. Dr. Mark continues: "The George Gershwin syndrome of the thirties is still being treated in the seventies. Recently eighteen patients were committed to a mental hospital at one of our best university centers who turned out to have tumors of their limbic brains. In some cases, the true nature of this illness was not recognized until the tumor had caused the patient's death."[11]

There is solid medical evidence linking aggressive behavior to focal brain disease. Such behavior, according to Mark, "is often present in such clinical disorders as temporal lobe epilepsy, temporal lobe tumors, infections of the brain (such as rabies and post-encephalitic syndromes), and serious brain injuries which affect the under-surfaces of the frontal lobes (usually a transient phenomenon in the last disorder)."[12]

We certainly do not want ever to arrive in our society at a point where the violence of political protesters, ghetto rioters, and others is "cured" by brain surgery. But neither can we discount the role of brain dysfunction in many instances of violent, aggressive behavior. Both the moral sensitivity and the diagnostic skill of the neurosurgeon are crucial in deciding in a particular case whether or not brain surgery is indicated.

Another practical problem lies in obtaining valid consent for psychosurgery. If the patient is unable to make a rational decision, his nearest relatives or someone else will have to make it for him. But since there is frequently a danger that the relatives or legal guardians will make their decision in their own best interest rather than that of the patient, many hospitals have set up review committees made up of psychiatrists, neurosurgeons, lawyers, clergymen, and lay persons.

If such a committee is to be set up, it should be composed of people who are professionally, economically, and psychologically independent of the physician whose case is being reviewed. The committee should make sure that all other less drastic measures have been tried and given a chance to work. And they should make their decision in the interest of the patient, not in the interest of the relatives, the hospital staff, society, the state, or the experimenting surgeon. Dr. Valenstein has further remarked: "All members of the review committee should hold the patient's interest as the foremost consideration, but it would be a good practice to have one member serve as the patient's ombudsman. It would be the ombudsman's specific responsibility to protect the patient by questioning in detail whether alternative therapies were sufficiently explored and also to determine if consent was given under conditions that assured the patient or guardian was maximally informed."[13]

Especially touchy is the case of prisoners. Some men are in prison, often in solitary confinement, because of aggressive and violent behavior due to brain dysfunction. But because it is extremely difficult to insure the prisoner's personal freedom, many people feel that as a practical rule we should never permit brain surgery to be performed on anyone in prison.

There is certainly a grave danger here that bears close monitoring. In fact, as a normal rule the presumption should always be against performing brain surgery on prisoners. But, on the other hand, proper consent can sometimes be obtained, and if this is the case, it would not seem right to deny prisoners with brain disease access to surgical treatment which would probably be of real benefit to them.

Finally, most neurosurgeons and writers on the topic say that psychiatric surgery should be done "only as a last resort." Other treatments should be tried first—for instance, prolonged psychotherapy, drug therapy, and limited shock treatment. This is easy enough to understand, but two qualifications must be made. Dr. Scoville reminds us, first, that "any extensive or long continued shock therapy may well be more destructive to brain function than are the new limited surgical operations."[14] Second, it can sometimes be dangerous to wait too long. Psychosurgery should be a last resort, but this does not mean that it is to be no more than a final heroic effort at a cure. If one delays too long, sometimes the turning point in effective therapy will have been passed.

Moral generalizations may be helpful, but in the last analysis the sound judgment and moral goodness and integrity of the doctor will be decisive. The International Code of Medical Ethics adopted by the General Assembly of the World Medical Association wisely reminds us: "As a stream cannot rise above its source, so a code cannot change a low-grade man into a high-grade doctor, but it can help a good man to be a better man and a more enlightened doctor. It can quicken and inform a conscience, but not create one."[15]

Appendices

APPENDIX A

Catholic Hospital Ethics:

The Report of the Commission on Ethical and Religious Directives for Catholic Hospitals Commissioned by the Board of Directors of the Catholic Theological Society of America

INTRODUCTION: CRISIS OVER HOSPITAL ETHICS

1. There are almost eight hundred Roman Catholic hospitals in the United States, housing almost one-third of all the privately owned hospital beds in the country. Catholic hospitals are not only unique in their historical origins and in their generous service to the American public; they are also distinguished by their code of ethics.

2. The *Ethical and Religious Directives for Catholic Health Facilities*[1]—also referred to as a "national code"[2]—is a collection of ethical and religious principles and precepts designed to serve as Catholic hospital policy in those dioceses where the local bishop adopts it for use. The revision of the *Directives*, approved by the Roman Catholic bishops of the United States in November 1971, left the earlier (1955) version virtually unchanged in spite of some very noteworthy medical, ethical, social, and theological

developments experienced in the intervening years. Consequently, the 1971 *Directives* have raised some serious conflicts for the Catholic Church, for the public, for Catholic theology, for many medical personnel, for individual bishops, and for the Catholic hospitals themselves.

3. The result has been no ordinary academic debate or ecclesiastical dispute. For while the *Directives* offer the security of a definite church policy for those troubled with administrative problems, allegiance to some of its restrictions in the unqualified fashion called for in its preamble frequently excludes the provision of certain medical and surgical procedures commonly admitted in other hospitals, significantly restricts the freedom of patients and physicians, and causes intolerable institutional problems, thus contributing to situations in which the termination of some Catholic health services has been unavoidable. There are ample signs indicating that conformity to the ethical and theological principles and presuppositions of the 1971 *Directives* may well lead to further Catholic relinquishment of health services and perpetuate the conflicts presently being experienced in Catholic hospitals over internal policy questions pertaining to medical ethics.

4. We take the position that Catholic sponsorship of hospitals and other health facilities can be an effective and important means of service even in the present critical circumstances; but we also believe that if this sponsorship is to continue in a way that will respect good morality while acknowledging the rights and dignity of all concerned, there must be certain changes in the attitudes and policies which have been taken in the name of ethics.

5. This report is not simply a commentary on the new *Directives,* nor does it undertake to analyze systematically each of the specific prescriptions contained in the *Directives,* for this would require a lengthy and detailed analysis of a great number of different topics. Further studies would be necessary to accomplish that. Instead, this report presents theological and ethical reflections on the major issues involved in the presuppositions of such a set of directives, as well as in its implementation. Any serious attempt to assess the meaning, function, and applicability

of a code of ethics for Catholic hospitals leads to a discovery of many major questions, few of which have received adequate theological attention:

6. Why should there be Catholic hospitals? What is the identity, accountability, and responsibility of the contemporary Catholic hospital in today's American society? What is the Catholic hospital as agent of moral decision making? What are and what should be the processes of decision making? What is the function of a code of ethics for a health care facility? Is it a tool for decision making or a list of ready-made decisions? To what degree can the ethics of a profession or the moral teachings of a church be "codified"? Who should be responsible for composing and interpreting a hospital's code of ethics—the local bishop? All the bishops of the country? Church laity? Patients within individual hospitals? Community lay hospital committees? Theologians? Physicians and other health care personnel? Hospital officials and personnel? To what kinds of problems should the code be directed? What is the moral binding power of the *Directives,* and is dissent from them possible? Is it possible to set limits to legitimate dissent?

7. We hope that this report: (*a*) will provide some helpful principles for hospital administrators, medical personnel, and others involved in decision making; (*b*) will contribute to the theological basis for a prompt and thorough revision of the new directives; (*c*) will encourage theologians, physicians, and others to do further theological and ethical studies on the topics touched upon briefly in this report; and (*d*) will serve as the basis for further discussion and debate on these important issues.[3]

PART I.
HOSPITAL ETHICS IN A PLURALIST SETTING

Catholic Hospitals: Moral Accountability

8. In recent years the Catholic hospital—like the practice of medicine itself—has been undergoing social, cultural, and legal changes which profoundly affect its identity, its moral accountability, and its moral responsibility.[4] In common with other nonprofit, voluntary hospitals, the Catholic hospital is experiencing

increasing involvement with the civic community, with public agencies, and with government; and it is also experiencing increasing limitations on its ownership and its scope of freedom before the law.

9. Because they serve the public at large and are supported by federal and state funds, Catholic hospitals serve the public interest and are accountable to the public in their day-to-day operation, e.g., through federal and state agencies and hospital associations. As Catholic hospitals enter relationships of liaison, cooperation, and merger, they become responsible to and/or co-responsible with other medical institutions. As Catholic facilities extend themselves increasingly into community health care programs, it becomes more imperative that they offer comprehensive health care services. On a national level, too, Catholic hospitals are cooperating with various health and social welfare agencies and associations, and this has led to joint programs designed to meet mutual needs. Furthermore, an increasingly substantial segment of the non-Catholic community plays an important role within the Catholic hospital itself: on the board of trustees, in management, on the medical staff, among other personnel, and among its patients.

10. In a word, the Catholic hospital has gradually been altered from a strictly private institution to a more pluralistic community health care facility operated under Catholic auspices, although the extent of a pluralist dimension varies widely from hospital to hospital. While the Catholic hospital may be church property ("ecclesiastical patrimony"), with a religious congregation or diocese retaining legal control over it, it is clear that this health facility is becoming a quasi-public, pluralistic institution with multiple social and moral accountability.

11. The preamble of the current *Directives* offers a defensive, ahistorical response to the pluralistic setting of today's Catholic hospitals. It seems to want to insulate the Catholic hospital by giving serious acknowledgement only to its "vertical accountability," which is operative solely within the private structures of what canon law calls an "ecclesiastical moral person" (the Catholic hospital). This model of accountability also presumes

that Catholic hospitals are univocally identifiable as Roman Catholic, particularly by their being held uniformly accountable to hospital authorities (such as hospital administrators) who, in this regard, are assumed to be acting as agents for ecclesiastical authorities (religious superiors and ultimately bishops) in the implementation of detailed medical-ethical policies established by the church hierarchy. This model of accountability does encourage the fulfillment of what may be called the "conscience demands" of the corporate moral person, but fails to take into account recent socioethical developments.

12. It would be appropriate to today's pluralist situation to acknowledge the model of "horizontal accountability" which is also operative in the very identity of Catholic hospitals. The Catholic hospital is no longer on a religious island. As it becomes increasingly involved with the civic community and other health care entities, it becomes more accountable to them, affords them more representation in the affairs of the Catholic health care facility, and takes on more responsibility for providing them with an atmosphere of freedom. Consequently, the Catholic hospital-as-moral-person has gradually experienced a change in its social identity and moral accountability. Because the contemporary description of its responsibility is due to its pluralist setting, its problems related to policy and ethics must be understood against the background of contemporary pluralism.

Pluralism As Ethical Context

13. The empirical fact of pluralism pervades every major dimension of our lives—intellectual, cultural, social, ethical, and religious—and it provides the context for today's healing ministry of the Church. We are now being challenged to determine what our response to pluralism should be—how we should articulate the impact our pluralist setting in America has on the mission of the Catholic hospital and on the way in which ethical norms for these hospitals should be explicated.

14. We believe that response should be positive in tone and substance—not because we are forced by legal requirements or financial necessities to submit to the consequences of pluralism,

but because contemporary Catholic teaching has shown us the way toward a positive evaluation of pluralism. Prior to Vatican II, official Catholic teaching regarded pluralism as an unfortunate situation which had to be tolerated at best and actively opposed if possible. This view placed Catholicism in a defensive position: guidelines of minimal cooperation governed our civil and religious postures as an institution, lest cooperation in a pluralist setting be taken to mean compromise of religious and ethical principles.

15. A significant development of doctrine took place, however, as pluralism came to be acknowledged in principle as a normative context for understanding the ministry of the Church and her institutions, opening the way for a corresponding difference in institutional practice. The teaching of Vatican II manifests this development of doctrine. The *Declaration on Religious Freedom*[5] not only recognizes the fact of pluralism but accepts it as the historical norm in which Catholic participation in society must be conceived. The *Decree on Ecumenism*[6] affirms the ecclesial reality of other churches and the possibility of learning from the theological and ethical insights developed within other Christian communities. The *Constitution on the Church in the Modern World*[7] affirms the solidarity of the Church with the pluralist world and the need for a mutual learning experience through continuous dialogue.

16. In brief, the principles of Catholic theology emerging from Vatican II call for something more than an attitude which views pluralism as a situation which should be denied acceptance institutionally and resisted operationally. There still lingers within the Church today a preference for reliance upon reinforced institutional policy for the purpose of preserving the complete integrity of all the institution's doctrine and ethical prescriptions against the 'onslaught' of a pluralist environment. Yet these conciliar documents seek to orient the Catholic community toward the development of ways in which we can both serve the message of the Gospel which has been handed down to us and minister, in the name of Christ, to the needs of today's mankind through full and active collaboration (which means neither compromise nor betrayal) in the world of our day.

The Pluralist Dilemma of Catholic Hospitals

17. The consequences of pluralism profoundly affect the very notion of our hospital ethics, for they raise the question: Can Catholic hospitals, on religious and ethical grounds, continue to justify the refusal of certain health services which are legally permitted, commonly accepted in the medical world, and, at least in some cases, not morally harmful according to the judgment of many prudent men?

18. The fundamental dilemma of today's Catholic hospitals is the fundamental dilemma of contemporary pluralism, for in today's pluralistic world there are competing signs of the times. Some push us to broaden our ethical conceptions and practices, while others challenge us to reassert our vision of life. Some pluralist aspects of hospital service, such as community involvement, urge us to be less restrictive of what is permitted in our hospitals; and on the other hand the desire to maintain an "institutional identity" based on certain convictions about the Church's teaching authority accounts for our refusal to condone some actions.

19. In trying to retain a Catholic identity through institutional ethical policies we may violate the rights of others, neglect or harm the social good, and force an abdication of Catholic institutional presence in the hospital world. On the other hand, in seeking to become thoroughly acceptable in a pluralistic world by maximizing the freedom of all parties concerned and by offering all the commonly accepted medical services, we may needlessly violate some important values enshrined in the institutional ethical code, lose a significant Catholic identity, and drift into tacit acceptance of secularist values.

20. To strike the needed balance is a delicate task requiring a deep understanding of why there should be a Catholic presence in the hospital world; an accurate, credible, and usable set of directives; an astute sense of policy making and decision making on the local level; and an ability to make discreet adaptation to the contemporary situation (which is the question of "cooperation"). These topics will be treated in the following paragraphs.

PART II.
CATHOLIC PRESENCE IN HEALTH CARE INSTITUTIONS

21. There is considerable concern today over the institutional identity of the Catholic hospital and the "visibility" of the health care apostolate, principally for four reasons: (*a*) the contemporary world of medicine and hospital care is making it necessary for Catholic hospitals to exercise a somewhat less autonomous stewardship over their facilities; (*b*) legal factors are affecting the very ownership of the Catholic hospital by creating a trend toward less corporate privacy; (*c*) there is a decrease in the membership of the religious congregations which sponsor Catholic hospitals; and (*d*) there is not agreement among the membership of the sponsoring religious congregations whether the emphasis of their health apostolate should be on "institutional management" or "personal witness." Consequently, the question is being asked: Why and how should the Church be involved in the apostolate of health care institutions, and how can it preserve its Christian and Catholic identity?

22. Catholic involvement in health care has deep religious and historical origins rooted in certain beliefs and expressed in service and witness. The apostolate to the sick, the suffering, and the dying has been one of the most distinguished, selfless, and tangible services rendered by the servant Church to mankind. Like the work of Christ himself, the Catholic Church's care of the sick and dying is ultimately directed to leading men to the Father. It witnesses to the healing mission of Christ, manifests his work of mercy and reconciliation, and at the same time provides an environment in which human values, such as the dignity of human life, may be more clearly perceived, appreciated, and appropriated.

23. This environment may be created by church institutions, but it is sustained primarily by the inner Christian dynamic of dedicated service to the physical, mental, and spiritual care of both Catholics and non-Catholics, especially to the poor, the neglected, and the abandoned. In particular, a pastoral concern for the spiritual welfare of the sick, the injured, and the

troubled should continue to be a distinguishing feature of our Christian witness and a unique kind of Christian presence in the work of maintaining and restoring health in Catholic facilities.

24. Christian acceptance of Christ's commission to care for the sick is adaptable to many forms, methods, and institutions, as history testifies. It is true that an important dimension of this apostolate of the Church has been its witness to a moral stability that survives the recurring espousal and rejection of values in many segments of society. Yet the Church has accomplished this moral stability through a diverse succession of institutions and in spite of a certain fluctuation in its own understanding of ethical norms.

25. In contemporary America, the Church's religious and ethical presence in hospital service (aside from the spiritual and pastoral presence mentioned above) may be accomplished on the institutional level, on the personal level, and overlapping these two categories, in a communitarian way. These kinds of presence are not necessarily mutually exclusive. The actual applicability and real impact of a set of ethical directives will vary according to the combination of these factors in an individual hospital.

26. Church agencies such as religious congregations and dioceses have sought to ensure the active presence of a "Catholic philosophy" in health care facilities through institutional sponsorship. Institutional presence may be effected by ownership and/or control. Hospital ownership by a church agency affords the greatest guarantee that official Catholic teaching will serve as codified hospital policy. Another means of accomplishing the religious and moral presence of the Church in this ministry in an institutional way is through the model of retaining policy control and control over decisions affecting the charter and bylaws of the hospital. According to this plan, the hospital assets are owned by another corporation, and a contract is arrived at with the religious congregation that operates the hospital, with the agreement that the hospital is to be operated according to the philosophy of the sponsoring group. Some believe that this model is a viable alternative, while others doubt that the

"Catholic code" could permanently continue to be institutional policy under this arrangement.

27. Institutional presence of whatever kind is not the only manner of Catholic presence in the hospital apostolate, and a Catholic presence that is only institutional without the dynamism of corporate dedication to moral values is not a religious and moral presence at all. In the absence of such corporate commitment, the adoption of a code would be an act of policy but not an ethical pursuit. If an institutional presence is to have a moral soul, there must simultaneously be a communal Catholic presence which both creates and asserts a Christian goal and purpose based on a religiously motivated covenant of moral values. The patients (for whom the hospitals should exist!) can be expected to benefit by this communal witness as they have in the past. Only if this witness is present will the hospital's code be able to serve an honest declaratory function to the larger community which it serves.

28. It would seem that the essential Christian contribution to health care is facilitated by, without being irrevocably tied to, ownership. Certainly the Church should never willingly abdicate all institutional witness in an area as important as health care. It is true that the autonomy of Catholic hospital ownership is being curtailed, and for some this threatens to place limitations on a distinctively Catholic style of codified and institutional ethical presence. This trend should caution us to reflect more seriously on several factors which, in our contemporary situation, highlight the importance of Catholic institutional presence in the health care field, specifically: (*a*) the consideration that a distinctive institutional presence makes it possible to influence and direct societal decisions regarding health care; and (*b*) the fact that, through its institutional presence, a voluntary association of dedicated Christians renders a community service through the investment of many of its resources, not the least of which is its communal witness. On the other hand, this same trend toward a lessened autonomy of the private hospital should move Catholic hospital personnel to a greater and more genuine communitarian witness to the

moral and ethical values involved in the care of the sick, and to strive to accomplish this in a way that goes beyond mere conformity to the moral prescripts of a code of ethics.

29. Certain aspects of hospital service are causing more emphasis to be placed nowadays on the personal level of Catholic presence in church-sponsored hospitals. In addition to the four general reasons mentioned in par. 21, two more specific causes could be indicated. (*a*) Responsibility for the affairs of the Catholic hospital is being placed more and more on the local institution itself, which is increasingly diversified in the make-up of its structures. This calls more attention to the individuals involved and raises the question whether they will accomplish an effective Catholic presence in a situation where, at least to some degree, they must compete with a multiplicity of interests (see par. 47 below). (*b*) At a time when impersonal mechanization and depersonalized programming are so much a part of health care, the need for the humanizing dimension of dedicated Christian service is greater than ever before. In fact this may well be the greatest ethical challenge for today's Catholic hospital. Personal concern and innovative programs relating directly to people's needs are required to counteract this tendency.

30. It is by no means the Catholic personnel alone (on the medical and nursing staffs, in the administration and on the board of trustees) who can make this kind of presence felt on a personal level. Individuals of any or no religious creed are also called upon—in an institution pluralistic in its make-up—to give a witness of concerned and personalized care. Yet the Catholic sponsored hospital should be uniquely prepared to give effective moral leadership to foster this personal kind of presence. Furthermore, personal witness is strongest where a community sense of dedication to values is strongest. The Catholic sponsored institution should have a special ability to assist in creating this communal experience which will support a goal-oriented personal witness on the part of personnel who otherwise may find themselves morally isolated in a depersonalized hospital system. Consequently, it should be an objective of

prime importance for the Catholic sponsored hospitals to develop within the individual facilities a community with those values which most surely support the Christian purpose of serving the sick.

31. The question of a Catholic presence—institutional, personal, and above all communal—is a crucial question if health care is to be seen as an extension of Christ's mission of mercy in a pluralistic setting. A unique Catholic presence is made both possible and imperative by the corporate moral convictions of the Church which should find their expression in the policy of a Catholic hospital. Yet a tenacious and insular conformity to a rigid code of ethics should not be appealed to as a means of "keeping Catholic health facilities Catholic" in the face of the social upheaval being experienced by these institutions. The other parts of this report suggest a broader context for the effective use of ethical directives in the accomplishment of this goal. An institutional code should reflect an awareness of why and how the institution will accomplish this presence and why individuals should want to look to the code for guidance in their personal and corporate moral witness. Educational and formative efforts should be made to develop an appreciation for this fundamental dimension of Christian medical ethics, for the benefit of those engaged in the work of Catholic sponsored as well as other health care facilities.

PART III. THE CODE AND ETHICAL DECISION MAKING

The Code in a Christian Context

32. In attempting to understand and interpret a code of ethics, several fundamental questions present themselves, viz.: What is the purpose of a code of ethics? What is its function in decision making? What is the purpose of a code in a Christian context? What is its role in the functioning of a Catholic hospital?

33. A code of ethics, whether professional or institutional, can have several purposes, all related to a group's evaluation of behaviour. It may be instructional (providing moral and ethical

information to the uninformed); declaratory (declaring the group's values, goals, and objectives to its own members and to others); conservative (upholding certain essential standards of behaviour which conserve the unity and identity of the group); policy setting (providing a definite method of action to guide and determine decisions and to evaluate behaviour once the decisions have been taken); arbitrational (enunciating principles and establishing or allowing for procedures for the resolution of conflicts of duties and conflicts of consciences); and/or coercive (creating varying degrees of social pressure or sanction so as to guarantee adherence to a certain ethical behaviour and to provide both internal and external identification). Briefly, a code is a statement of values, an assertion of goals, and/or an expression of rules whose purposes all focus on good decision making and behaviour.

34. The U. S. bishops' "national code" seeks to fulfill most of these purposes. It must be noted, however, that the "group" whose values is being declared and conserved should not be solely the hierarchical "teachers of morality," but the entire group of all those involved in this endeavor.

35. How does a code relate to decision making? This depends partly on how the statement of a code is expressed, for a codified statement or the expression of a directive may be either a *moral prescription* or an *ethical principle.* A moral prescription either forbids or commands specific behaviour, usually in an all-inclusive or negative formulation, such as: "Sterilization, whether permanent or temporary, for men or for women, may not be used as a means of contraception" (*Directives,* par. 18). An ethical principle, on the other hand, is a statement—usually in the form of a positive formulation—of the group's understanding of values related to a certain kind of human behaviour. It emphasizes general values, but not to the exclusion of specific rules of conduct, for example: "Because the ultimate personal expression of conjugal love in the marital act is viewed as the only fitting context for the human sharing of the divine act of creation, donor insemination and insemination that is totally artificial are morally objectionable" (*Directives,* par. 21).

36. These two kinds of directives play different roles in decision making, depending on norms of interpretation. Moral prescriptions are generally understood as requirements which hold those bound by it to a predetermined behaviour pattern, and consequently tend to be a list of decisions before the fact. They leave little room for interpretation of circumstances, rules, or values. Ethical principles, on the other hand, are not so much a list of ready-made decisions as they are a set of guidelines which provide structure and illumination for judgment concerning specific behaviour.

37. A hospital code of ethics should necessarily include both types of directives. The U. S. bishops' *Directives* contain both types, but place by far the greater emphasis on moral prescriptions. Yet many of their prohibitions do call for some degree of further interpretation and application, particularly those which are qualified by such factors as intention or consent, as in any type of case where the distinction of "direct" and "indirect" has customarily been made. Thus the prohibition of sterilization would be an instance of a moral prescription which is not in every respect a decision before the fact, for further decisions must be made concerning those sterilizations which in fact should not be prohibited.

38. When a code is used in a Christian institution established for the care of the sick and dying, it is qualified by certain additional characteristics. In this case the code partially expresses the Christian group's vision of the vocation of healing and establishes certain structures which enable the hospital to accomplish and perfect its role of care for the human person. The moral and ethical standards which this institution affirms are understood as partaking in the law of healing which the whole Church seeks to follow in faithful extension of the healing Christ. Moral standards for the Catholic hospital should be looked upon the same way that moral law is viewed in a Christian perspective. The moral law is not held principally to be a legal enactment, codified and promulgated with penalties imposed, for the law of the Christian is Christ himself in whom we have life and who is therefore the law of our lives. For the Christian

the moral law is not conceived primarily as a restrictive force but as a liberating force. Its function is to guide and inform Christian love and hence Christian compassion, care, and healing; and to aid conscientious judgments in an atmosphere of freedom.

39. A number of important elements which constitute a Christian theology of moral law are unfortunately lacking in the preamble of the U.S. bishops' *Directives*, which offers a predominantly legalistic dimension to the directives. A very different theological explanation is found in the preamble to the Canadian Catholic *Medico-Moral Guide*, which also adds: "The Guidelines . . . should be read and understood not as commands imposed from without, but as demands of the inner dynamism of the human and Christian life. . . . (T)heir application to a particular situation will usually entail a great deal of prudence and wisdom. . . . The Guidelines should serve to enlighten the judgment of conscience. They cannot replace it."[8] The differences between the underlying theological presuppositions of the U.S. and Canadian hierarchies in reference to the purpose and function of a set of directives in medical ethics account for the charge of "geographic morality" which is becoming a common cause of consternation among North American Catholics who are concerned with health care institutions and services.

The Code and Magisterial Pronouncements

40. The U.S. *Directives* are not a comprehensive professional code nor simply a set of guidelines as described above. They are predominantly a statement of institutional policy indicating what must not be done by medical personnel if they are to be admitted to practice medicine in Catholic sponsored health care facilities. These policies are mostly moral norms either taken from or directly supported by papal moral teachings. As such, they are a selective collection of assertions from authoritative, magisterial teachings.

41. Magisterial teachings should call forth deep respect and sincere adherence on the part of Catholics. Yet these teachings do not all enjoy the same degree of certitude and binding

power, and none of the concrete norms in the *Directives* is infallible. In particular, there is no longer any good reason (if there ever was one) for concealing the fact of the greater and lesser degrees of certitude enjoyed by official church teachings in moral matters. Magisterial teaching itself acknowledges this variety, and intelligent men and women today can easily see that not all the actions prohibited by the 1971 *Directives* are "clearly wrong" in an undifferentiated way as proposed by the U.S. bishops. Today's situation of pluralism in particular should prod us to more openness and candor, both in acknowledging what can be permitted on occasion even in the face of a general prohibition which the Catholic community is reluctant to abandon, and in firmly supporting the prohibitions of which we are deeply convinced and which seem to strike more deeply to the roots of our faith identity. Simply to repeat past magisterial pronouncements does not suffice. Constant scrutiny and wise discretion are required if ecclesiastical moral pronouncements are to be transformed into good hospital policy.

42. A "code" of medical ethics which relies on magisterial pronouncements will require certain precautions and clarifications, several of which are not apparent in the present code. There can be a great distance between the historical and cultural context, the authorship and style of the papal teaching on the one hand, and the world of contemporary Catholic hospital problems on the other hand. If the directives are to be effective, this gap must be bridged: the unaltered, precise words of a pope cannot guarantee relevancy to a highly professional world. Since a set of institutional directives can scarcely be an effective tool for medical decision making if it is not rightly understood, some principles of interpretation and criteria for the resolution of conflicts must be included. The new *Directives* are particularly remiss in this regard. In spite of very extensive magisterial and theological developments since 1955 in the area of law, conscience, and freedom, the new *Directives* are more insistent on the certitude and binding power of the norms than the previous *Directives* were. The following important principle for the resolution of doubt, which was contained in the 1955 edition,

has been omitted in the 1971 edition: "In questions legitimately debated by theologians, liberty is left to physicians to follow the opinions which seem to them more in conformity with the principles of sound medicine."[9] That practical principle expressed the notion of freedom in cases of doubt; and because that freedom should still be in effect today, the statement of the 1955 edition is still valid for moral decision making, but with two qualifications: (a) the "questions legitimately debated by theologians" are now considerably extended, for they may now include questions which have previously been pronounced upon by popes; and (b) the "liberty" spoken of should not be seen as exclusively or even primarily that enjoyed by the physician, for it is the patient who has the first and most basic responsibility to make decisions on his own behalf.

43. Furthermore, ethical directives must make a clear delineation between general principles and their application in more specific rules; should acknowledge that some principles deal with "hard cases" where it is not always clear what may be done; and should indicate whether a prohibition is only given as an instance of a more general and more important principle which it is intended to illustrate (which might explain, for instance, par. 21 of the *Directives*).

44. It may be necessary in some instances to single out for firm affirmation as hospital policy a moral norm derived from official church pronouncements or from theological reflection. A particularly grave threat to deep human values may make this necessary. There is, for example, a vast difference between the values involved in the prohibitions of "masturbation as a means of obtaining seminal specimens" (par. 21) and "directly intended destruction of a viable fetus" (par. 12). The fact that both prohibitions are taught by the magisterium does not make them equally grave, nor does the fact that neither is infallible make them equally unimportant. The principles of dissent, which will be referred to more extensively below, have their limits; and today's situation of pluralism as described above urges us to support certain standards more strongly than others lest our more fundamental moral values—those more surely related to

a Gospel-based understanding of man—be lost. To maintain this moral identity it may be necessary to prohibit some behaviour more fully in a policy statement and in application than could be sustained in given instances through ethical reflection alone. We believe that this approach to the establishment of an institutional code—in its "declaratory," "conservative," and "policy setting" functions—is fully warranted in reference to abortion. The field of medicine in particular and society in general, by extending the "indications" for abortion or removing any need for such indications, are admitting abortion on demand, which ought to be opposed on ethical and social grounds by Catholic institutions. The fact that society is abandoning other means of protecting human life itself at its earlier stages of development makes even more urgent a general but clear and firm policy of exclusion of abortion on the part of Catholic health institutions.

Decision Making: A Shared Responsibility

45. The existence of a truly adequate code will not provide all the needed direction in ethical questions. Three sorts of problems arise calling for further discernment. (*a*) Code and policy must be interpreted, to establish, for example, whether exceptions can be made, such as in shared facilities or joint practices. (*b*) Working policies must be developed to provide for cases not clearly covered in the code or other policy. (*c*) Decisions must be made in individual cases, to determine, for instance, what can be done in emergency situations or in "hard cases." Many of these questions are highly particularized for individual Catholic hospitals, and those faced with such questions should not lightly abdicate their prime responsibility to make judgments on moral principles as applied to medical and health care problems. In fact, these decisions are being made daily in our Catholic health facilities.

46. It would be mistaken to think that medical-ethical decisions can simply be referred to some other agency such as the local bishop. The preamble of the new *Directives* states that debated questions in medical ethics "must be finally submitted to the teaching authority of the Church in the person of the

local bishop, who has the ultimate responsibility for teaching Catholic doctrine." This unqualified statement of the local bishop's competence in medical ethics has been questioned on theological grounds, on legal-medical grounds, and for reasons of common sense. In any event, the bishop is rarely consulted; and when he is consulted he frequently appeals to a theologian who is competent to give an ethical reply. This pattern of referral seems to amount to an acknowledgment of the principle of consultation in practice if not in stated policy. Although the bishop should not be considered the sole ultimate authority in the field of medical ethics and should not be cast into the role of final consultant in the treatment of a patient, this does not imply that the moral authority of the Church should be jeopardized, or that the bishop has no leadership role to play. Certainly the formulation of local hospital policy should not be made in isolation from the whole Church or from the hierarchical Church. This unity of local policy with the Church at large can be accomplished in several ways; but certainly the teaching of the local bishop who is in communion with the whole Church is an important factor. By his word he makes the power of the healing Christ present in a unique way. Furthermore, due to peculiar local circumstances, some of the decisions taken in hospitals can have pastoral significance for the diocese as a whole, thus involving the interests of the episcopal office. The ministry of Catholic hospitals has more to gain today than ever before from the enlightened leadership of the local bishop because of the way in which health care service participates both in secular society and in the life of the Church.

47. In fact, however, both moral and legal responsibility for Catholic hospitals is being focused more and more on the structure of the local institution: its board of trustees, its administration, and its medical staff. Giving the local health care facility more autonomy is more appropriate to the notion of shared responsibility within the Church and more in conformity with the principle of subsidiarity. The same principle of subsidiarity may indicate in some instances that certain key decisions affecting the total hospital involvement of the entire sponsoring

group (the religious congregation) should be relegated to the decision makers of the sponsoring or corporate group, thus determining in advance some of the institutional policy for many Catholic hospitals. Even so, many decisions will consistently and most appropriately be those of the local institutions where the basic task of decision making resides. Many important decisions, including policy decisions, should rightly be made at the local level because of the increasingly complex nature of the questions arising in medicine today and the need for special competence in responding to them as they arise in individual cases. Thus, the complex responsibility of ethical decision making goes beyond without nullifying the "national code" which seeks to establish a uniform national list of ethical and religious standards. Some procedures are needed at the local level to facilitate proper consultation among those who are the principal moral agents: the patient, the physician, medical staff, administrative staff, and others.

48. Various parties should be involved in the decision making process, so as to draw on appropriate competencies according to the complexity of the case. It is difficult to state—in reference to varying hospital situations and varying categories of problems to be solved—precisely which competencies should be represented. They might include some combination of the following: physicians, members of the medical staff, nurses, medical social workers, department heads, administrators, ethicists, and those holding pastoral positions (bishop, parish priest, or chaplain). The key party in these decisions is the patient; and, depending on the kind of decision to be made, spokesmen representing the civic communities which the hospital serves should also be included. The principle involved is that of broad consultation, so that all those with a direct claim in the decision to be made may be permitted and encouraged to share in the decision. In some instances this should be accomplished more formally as, for example, through a committee; in other instances, less formally. It would seem, however, that some of the policy questions listed above would best be handled through an ethics committee, at least for purposes of seeking recommendations.

Medico-moral committees (whether institutional or inter-institutional or both) could fill an essential need for the solution of cases, serve as a means of exercising and enhancing the moral agency of the hospital as a corporate moral person, foster continuing education in medical ethics, and provide a much needed structure for a continuing revision of the present *Directives*.

49. Some working principles are important for hospital decision making which involves the code and multiple moral agency. The central agency of the patient must be acknowledged and his freedom should be maximized, though not to the exclusion of other considerations. The patient has the right to the fullest amount of information (medical and ethical) necessary for informed and responsible consent, and often he has the right to determine medical practice in his regard on the basis of his consent or dissent—but this latter right is not without limit. (See par. 44 above and pars. 52 and 63 below.)

PART IV. CONSCIENCE AND THE *DIRECTIVES*

The Directives and Religious Liberty

50. The foregoing sections on the meaning of the *Directives* and the problems of institutional decision making only take on their full meaning in the context of individual decision making where the role of conscience comes into play. Against the background of Part I of this report, the question arises: How does the context of pluralism affect the application of our ethical norms? Or, more specifically, must non-Catholic physicians and patients conform totally to the Catholic code of ethics in spite of their own sincere convictions of conscience to the contrary if they choose or are forced by circumstances to make use of a Catholic health facility which serves a pluralistic community?

51. The normative framework governing this relationship is the right to religious liberty, which means that no one is to be coercively constrained into belief or action contrary to his own convictions; and conversely that no one is to be coercively re-

strained by civil power from action (worship, witness, practice) according to his convictions. The dictates of this right should be applied analogously to the realm of Catholic hospital practice, with implications particularly for non-Catholic patients and staff.

52. The non-Catholic patient enjoys the right to religious liberty. In his case, as in the case of all men, the basis of the right is the dignity of the patient as person. The exercise of this right cannot be absolute; it is limited: (*a*) by the patient's responsibility to seek competent professional advice; (*b*) by the need to protect the rights of other innocent persons; (*c*) by the patient's obligation to respect his own duties toward others; and (*d*) by his obligation not to disturb the public order (or the larger social good) disproportionately.[10]

53. The basis for extending the right to religious freedom into questions of professional practice is the expertise enjoyed by professionals; and the implication of this application is that physicians have both a right and a duty to follow their well-formed conscience in the treatment of patients. The exercise of this right is limited, even outside of church-sponsored institutions, by the personal and social responsibilities mentioned in par. 52. These limitations may be expressed: (*a*) by society at large through the law; (*b*) by peers through professional ethics; and (*c*) by patient's giving or withholding of consent.

54. The critical question is whether the exercise of the right of religious liberty should be limited also by the fact of administering or seeking treatment in a Catholic hospital. From the hospital's perspective the issue is whether it can allow a course of action dictated by the conscience of the patient, or of both the patient and the physician, but contrary to the professed institutional code (or institutional "conscience") of the hospital. If the hospital invariably insists on the execution of its moral norms, it will presumably be acting according to its own moral standards, but it may also be disproportionately infringing on the rights of other people in our society. The moral principles governing the resolution of this conflict, whether on the institutional or the personal level, are the principles of "cooperation."

55. The theology of cooperation has varied according to pro-

gressively different cultural and religious views on the relation of the Catholic to the world around him. Today a theology of cooperation must be formulated and interpreted in light of the church's affirmation of the right of religious liberty, its acceptance of pluralism in principle, and its teaching of ethical norms with varying degrees of affirmation according to a scale of moral values. Coordinating these three elements is not a simple task: it is more a task of the prudential art of Christian living than of theological speculation. Norms, no matter how detailed, cannot supply the answers. To arrive at decisions concerning cooperation requires a good ethical sense, consultation with those directly involved, and a knowledge of the local situation. Also helpful is an understanding of the working principles of a theology of cooperation.

56. Traditionally, the principles governing "cooperation in evil" sought to solve problems associated with the permitted degree of cooperation in another person's action which was taught and presumed to be morally evil. The degree of "material cooperation" tolerated was relative, for it involved a balancing of good and evil effects and took account of degrees of necessity for permitting the action itself. In today's circumstances, and particularly since the more recent development of the doctrine of religious liberty, the question of "cooperation" is not simply whether one may participate in the (presumably objectionable) *act* of another, but whether one may cooperate with another *person* who may or may not have a right to engage in certain actions. Consequently, a correct understanding of cooperation (which cannot be extensively elaborated in this report) should be broadened so as to take into account the following criteria which refer to the individual and the institution, and which have taken on special ethical significance in recent times: (*a*) assuring the fulfillment of the individual's right to adequate medical care; (*b*) protecting the right to religious liberty; (*c*) avoiding scandal in the sense of true moral harm in a pluralistic setting; and (*d*) being aware of the changed significance of moral agency and moral responsibility. This latter point will now be explained in the context of today's Catholic hospital.

57. Medical technology and medical resources have made medical services more available. However, these advances have been accomplished through a restructuring of medical services and institutions in such a way that those engaged in delivering these services now frequently enjoy fewer options and less autonomy in the performance of their essential work. Consequently, the reality of a more highly organized *functional* cooperation in health care delivery frequently shifts the *ethical* question of cooperation from the person-to-person level where it was previously almost exclusively seen (the doctor-patient relationship) to levels involving larger groups and even entire institutions. Examples of this would be shared facilities among hospitals and group medical practices.

58. These changes in the moral agency, i.e., in the way in which different parties are responsible for the medical, surgical, or health care actions, signify that pluralism is more than a context: it has inherently affected the very meaning of the actions, and this in turn affects the degree of "cooperation" which can be permitted (without, of course, deliberately consenting to a moral disvalue). Catholics in a pluralist country have long been "cooperating" in collective actions which have moral effects at the social level which they would not want to initiate from their own moral conscience. We suggest that Catholic physicians in group practices and Catholic hospitals involved in shared facilities (to mention but two examples), where they do not have autonomous control over what happens in these collective situations, may operate under comparable principles of cooperation according to the criteria set forth above. The actual determination of what can be permitted by way of "cooperation" and still be within the scope of the hospital's responsibilities will depend very much on circumstances which alter the scope of the hospital's responsibilities in reference to the rights of the patient. For instance, it may be necessary to permit a procedure in a Catholic hospital which is the community's only health facility, while the same action would not have to be admitted in a Catholic hospital located in a large metropolitan area where other facilities are available. Medical

or surgical treatment may be morally permissible in an emergency situation where a delay might involve grave risks, while the same kind of treatment may be excluded in elective situations.

The Directives and the Right of Dissent

59. The normative framework governing the relationship of the conscience of the Catholic to official church pronouncements contained in the *Directives* is the teaching of the Church on freedom of conscience and on the right of legitimate dissent.

60. Conscience provides man with a personal and concrete moral dictate concerning what is to be done and what is to be avoided. It cannot be the sole arbiter of truth nor is it a law unto itself. It must be formed through openness to the Spirit in love and through docility to objective moral norms. However, once the dictate of conscience is prepared for in mind and in heart and is perceived with sufficient moral certainty, it provides the ultimate norm of moral conduct and must be obeyed even if erroneous. "In all his activity, man is bound to follow his conscience faithfully, in order that he may come to God for whom he was created."[11]

61. The hierarchical teaching office of the Catholic Church has asserted its authority to teach in the area of "faith and morals," even though the precise meaning of these terms, especially the term "moral," has never been clearly defined. The moral norms of medical ethics taught by the authoritative, papal, and hierarchical magisterium—no matter how specific and clear these teachings may be—are not infallible, nor do they require the full acceptance of an act of faith on the part of Catholics. They call for a "religious assent," the precise nature of which is still very much debated among theologians. It should involve reverential acknowledgment of the (papal) teaching office and "sincere adherence" to the pope's judgments, "according to his manifest mind and will."[12]

62. The reactions of bishops, theologians, and laity to the papal encyclical *Humanae vitae* have more firmly than ever established the right of dissent from such papal teaching when there are sufficient reasons for so doing. Consequently, to uphold

the "right of dissent" is a position that is theologically supportable and definitely within the pale of the Roman Catholic faith commitment.

63. Following these developments within the Church, it may safely be stated that moral decision makers affected by the new U.S. *Directives*—principally patients and physicians, but not excluding administrative and medical staff, as well as ethical advisors of the foregoing (clergy and chaplains, for example)—may, in individual cases and on moral grounds, licitly act contrary to the concrete (and hence noninfallible) ethical directives, provided: (*a*) the decision is seriously arrived at in good conscience after careful reflection; (*b*) respectful and open-minded attention is paid to the authoritative teaching of the hierarchy, as well as other sources of moral wisdom, in the light of the Gospel; (*c*) no undue harm is done to the life, well-being, or rights of a third party; and (*d*) scandal is avoided. This last condition means that precautions must be taken to prevent this exception from causing more harm than good, so as not to significantly and unnecessarily hinder the community role of the Catholic health facility and the moral welfare of others.

64. Beyond the four conditions mentioned, the obvious theoretical limit to legitimate dissent is the truth itself as expressed in the reasons for the dissent from a particular teaching. The discussion among theologians who are freely and responsibly carrying out their function and in dialogue with people in the medical profession can serve as an indication of the practical limits of dissent. As mentioned above (par. 44), the limits to dissent should be taken very seriously, particularly for societal reasons. The total Catholic community has not reflected seriously enough on what the limits to dissent should be on specific questions (such as sterilization, for example), so as to protect the rights of innocent people (particularly the disadvantaged) and to preserve public order (see pars. 52-54 above). Further multi-disciplinary studies on these matters are urgently needed. Because both the basis for dissent and the need for limits to dissent are valid and important, and because policy guidelines—whatever they may be—should be taken seriously,

Catholic hospital directives need to be devised which will take both kinds of factors into account. Otherwise they will either be exaggerated or ignored, and both of these extreme consequences should be avoided at all costs.

Additional Recommendations

65. We recommend research by theologians, ethicists, medical scientists, and physicians, jointly when possible, on many of the topics touched upon throughout this report. High priority should be placed on this research.

66. Just as inferior medical training or inadequate hospital management will produce poor hospital service, a lack of knowledge and appreciation of the ethics of medicine and health care can lead to bad policy and harmful decisions. Education in medical ethics should be promoted within individual Catholic sponsored institutions and on a diocesan or regional basis.

67. We urge that steps be taken toward a prompt revision of the 1971 *Directives*. Procedures should be established for a thorough and systematic revision, which should involve all of the pertinent competencies.

68. It does not seem to be in conformity with the function of a code of ethics for Catholic hospitals that it should take into account the more perplexing ethical questions on the frontiers of bio-medical research, except insofar as they relate to medical and hospital practice. However, experimentation in these areas may indeed relate to hospital ethics. The Church should be more actively involved in ethical research into the newer questions of bioethics.

69. In the present *Directives*, questions related to sex and reproduction have received too much emphasis. More stress should be placed on the positive aspects of responsible parenthood. It should also be noted that a substantial number of Catholic theologians believes that there can be legitimate dissent from several of the specific paragraphs in the recently promulgated code, including the following: the condemnations of contraception, direct sterilization, masturbation for seminal analysis, and artificial insemination with the husband's seed;

the processes forbidden in the handling of extrauterine pregnancies; and the distinction between direct and indirect which is stated in terms of physical structure of the act itself. Each of these topics deserves more research and extensive dialogue within the Church.

70. The following are some topics that require more attention than has heretofore been given them in the ethics of Catholic health care facilities: (*a*) the Catholic hospital's service to the poor and underprivileged; (*b*) the ethics of power in the Catholic hospital, especially as this relates to the control over medical services by the medical profession, the "consumer," for example, and the determination of fees; (*c*) quality of health care in Catholic institutions as an ethical issue; (*d*) racial segregation and discrimination; (*e*) a just family wage, educational and career advancement opportunities, and the other benefits which can rightly be expected from employment in Catholic health facilities; (*f*) clearer guidelines on the right to die in dignity, the prolongation of human life, the definition of "extraordinary means" for preserving life, the ethics of medical heroics and the understanding of death as part of life; (*g*) the importance of obtaining informed consent and the efforts required on the part of the professionals involved; (*h*) transplantation: informed consent, use of children as donors; (*i*) human experimentation: safeguards, informed consent, use of children in experimentation; (*j*) genetic counselling: its necessity, its limitations, limits on "right to procreate" vs. freedom of choice; (*k*) the extent of the rights of the retarded to be cared for in a manner commensurate with their needs.

COMMISSION ON CATHOLIC HOSPITAL ETHICS[13]

Warren T. Reich, Chairman	Margaret A. Farley, R.S.M.
George D. Shoup, S.J.	Charles E. Curran
Robert H. Springer, S.J.	André E. Hellegers, M.D.
James A. O'Donohoe	George A. Kanoti
J. Bryan Hehir	Kieran Nolan, O.S.B.

August 1972.

APPENDIX B

The Medico-Moral Guide of Canadian Bishops

Preamble

This Medico-Moral Guide replaces the Moral Code used by the Association since 1955. The rapid evolution of the position of Canadian Catholic hospitals, medical progress, and the contemporary renaissance in Catholic moral thinking have sharply focused, particularly in recent times, the need for an updating of the previous Moral Code.

The reader will note the new title. The thinking of contemporary moralists and the aspirations of the Christian conscience seem to require this. A code refers to the law of a given society. It implies promulgation by legislative authority, the imposition of penalties upon those who disobey its commands, and even a coercive power to force compliance with its demands. But Christian moral life may not be viewed solely from the point of formal enactment of law and not even primarily from the standpoint of the imperative of the divine will. With such an approach, one cannot grasp the basic meaning of Christian moral life. There is indeed a law of moral life. The law of the Christian is Christ himself in whom we have life and therefore also the law of our life. The exigencies of the human person and of the new being in Christ extend to the whole realm of human life.

The Guidelines present a concise statement of these exigencies in the field of hospital work. They should be read and understood not as commands imposed from without, but as demands of the inner dynamism of human and Christian life. And precisely because they are that, their application to a particular situation will usually entail a great deal of prudence and wisdom. There, then, personal conscience will find its field of competence. The Guidelines should serve to enlighten this judgment of conscience. They cannot replace it.

In certain complex situations, and owing as much to the difficulty as to the importance of the decision, personal conscience will benefit from the opinions of specialists.

The Guidelines therefore propose the appointment of medico-moral committees whose work should be particularly important for the solution of concrete cases and for the continuing revision of the present Guidelines.

I. *General Norms*

Art. 1. The following provisions are for the guidance of medical and administrative staffs and patients in Catholic hospitals. They should also be a guide to Catholics working in other Canadian hospitals.

Art. 2. The Catholic hospital should be a privileged place for the activity of the Saving Christ and for the extension of his spirit among men. By his concern for human infirmity, his sensitivity to human suffering, his respect for the human person, and his zealous will to free man from his burdens, the Christian —in the likeness of Christ—will show anxious concern to be for all men a witness of the "good news" of salvation and an instrument of the grace of the Kingdom.

Art. 3. Every person must respect the dictates of the conscience of a patient.

Art. 4. No person is obliged to take part in a medical activity which he judges in conscience to be immoral.

Art. 5. A medico-moral committee should be set up in each conference of the CHAC or in each member association of the CHAC and, when advisable, in the hospital itself.

Art. 6. Such a committee should normally consist of at least five members, two of whom should be doctors and two theologians. This representation of doctors and theologians should be retained in the event of increase in the committee membership. The committee should not neglect to obtain the advice of a specialist in the medical field of the case under consideration by the committee.
Art. 7. When doubt exists in the mind of the doctor, patient, or administrator, as to the application of these Guidelines to a particular case, or when the Guidelines do not appear to cover the particular case, the doctor should submit the case to the medico-moral committee for study and recommendation. The recommendation of the committee should serve as a guideline for the particular case submitted for consultation.
Art. 8. When an emergency case exists and the committee is unable to meet, the person to whom such responsibility has been delegated by the competent authority in the hospital should make the final decision. He should normally consult with a theologian and then present a report of the case and his decision to the committee.

II. The Right to Life

Art. 9. Every human being has a right to live, and every effort should be made to protect that right.
Art. 10. However, man is not bound to have recourse to every means to prolong life. Neither the patient nor the doctor is obligated to resort to involved techniques for artificial survival.
Art. 11. Euthanasia is a form of homicide; it is forbidden. To neglect ordinary means to prolong life is equivalent to euthanasia.
Art. 12. Any medical intervention that would cause death (autopsy, taking a heart for transplant, etc.) may be done only when death is certified.
Art. 13. From the moment of conception life must be guarded with the greatest care. All deliberate medical action, the purpose of which is to deprive a foetus or an embryo of its life, is immoral.
Art. 14. However, medical means required to cure a grave

illness in a pregnant woman, and which cannot be deferred until the foetus is viable, are allowed even though it might endanger the pregnancy in progress.

III. The Right to Bodily Integrity

Art. 15. Man has the right to the integrity of his body as well as that of his bodily functions.

Art. 16. Surgical operations are morally justified only if the good to be derived by the patient is in proportion to the grievousness of the foreseeable resultant damage; this good can only be normally that of the patient.

Art. 17. However, the giving of blood, a skin graft, a bone membrane, one organ of a pair is allowed for the well-being of another person. In transplants it is also lawful to make use of organs taken from corpses.

Art. 18. Sterilization, whether permanent or temporary, for man or for woman, may not be used as a means of birth control.

Art. 19. "Also to be rejected is any procedure, whether in preparation for the act of marriage, or while the act is being carried out, or as it is proceeding to its natural goals, which aims at blocking procreation either as an end desired, or as means to some other end" (*Humanae Vitae*, 14).

N.B. Reference should be made to the Canadian bishops' documents on the pastoral application of this general direction.

Art. 20. Morally, the conjugal act is necessary for procreation. Insemination that is totally artificial is immoral. However, help may be given to a normally performed conjugal act to attain its purpose.

IV. The Patient Has Also Other Rights

Art. 21. Man has a right that his body and person be treated with respect no matter how disabled they may be.

Art. 22. Medical secrets must remain inviolable. In case of necessity, and with the consent at least legitimately presumed of the patient, such a secret may be revealed to those having a right to know.

Art. 23. Every patient has a right to the proper medical care he needs.

Art. 24. At least, the reasonably presumed consent of the patient or of those having this right, is necessary for all medical and surgical treatment.

Art. 25. The patient has a right to be informed of his condition. This right becomes more urgent as his condition becomes more serious.

Art. 26. Those in charge should always be ready to see that patients in a hospital receive the necessary spiritual care.

9 April 1970

APPENDIX C

Ethical and Religious Directives for Catholic Health Facilities Issued By the United States Bishops

Preamble

Catholic health facilities witness to the saving presence of Christ and His Church in a variety of ways: by testifying to transcendent spiritual beliefs concerning life, suffering, and death; by humble service to humanity and especially to the poor; by medical competence and leadership; and by fidelity to the Church's teaching while ministering to the good of the whole person.

The total good of the patient, which includes his higher spiritual as well as his bodily welfare, is the primary concern of those entrusted with the management of a Catholic health facility. So important is this, in fact, that if an institution could not fulfill its basic mission in this regard, it would have no justification for continuing its existence as a Catholic health facility. Trustees and administrators of Catholic health facilities should understand that this responsibility affects their relationship with every patient, regardless of religion, and is seriously binding in conscience.

A Catholic sponsored health facility, its board of trustees and administration face today a serious difficulty as, with community support, the Catholic health facility exists side by side with other medical facilities not committed to the same moral code, or stands alone as the one facility serving the community. However, the health facility identified as Catholic exists today and serves the community in a large part because of the past dedication and sacrifice of countless individuals whose lives have been inspired by the Gospel and the teachings of the Catholic Church.

And just as it bears responsibility to the past, so does the Catholic health facility carry special responsibility for the present and future. Any facility identified as Catholic assumes with this identification the responsibility to reflect in its policies and practices the moral teachings of the Church, under the guidance of the local bishop. Within the community the Catholic health facility is needed as a courageous witness to the highest ethical and moral principles in its pursuit of excellence.

The Catholic sponsored health facility and its board of trustees, acting through its chief executive officer, further, carry an overriding responsibility in conscience to prohibit those procedures which are morally and spiritually harmful. The basic norms delineating this moral responsibility are listed in these Ethical and Religious Directives for Catholic Health Facilities. It should be understood that patients and those who accept board membership, staff appointment or privileges, or employment in a Catholic health facility will respect and agree to abide by its policies and these directives. Any attempt to use a Catholic health facility for procedures contrary to these norms would indeed compromise the board and administration in its responsibility to seek and protect the total good of its patients, under the guidance of the Church.

These directives prohibit those procedures which, according to present knowledge, are recognized as clearly wrong. The basic moral absolutes which underlie these directives are not subject to change, although particular applications might be modified as scientific investigation and theological development open up new problems or cast new light on old ones.

In addition to consultations among theologians, physicians, and other medical and scientific personnel in local areas, the Committee on Health Affairs of the United States Catholic Conference, with the widest consultation possible, should regularly receive suggestions and recommendations from the field, and should periodically discuss any possible need for an updated revision of these directives.

The moral evaluation of new scientific developments and legitimately debated questions must be finally submitted to the teaching authority of the Church in the person of the local Bishop, who has the ultimate responsibility for teaching Catholic doctrine.

The Ethical and Religious Directives for Catholic Health Facilities, dated September 1971, have been approved by the Committee on Doctrine of the National Conference of Catholic Bishop's (letter from Chairman, dated 30 October 1971). In the judgment of the Committee on Doctrine these Directives contain nothing contrary to Catholic teaching or morality.[1]

SECTION I: ETHICAL AND RELIGIOUS DIRECTIVES

General Directive

1. The procedures listed in these directives as permissible require the consent, at least implied or reasonably presumed, of the patient or his guardians. This condition is to be understood in all cases.
2. No person may be obliged to take part in a medical or surgical procedure which he judges in conscience to be immoral; nor may a health facility or any of its staff be obliged to provide a medical or surgical procedure which violates their conscience or these directives.
3. Every patient, regardless of the extent of his physical or psychic disability, has a right to be treated with a respect consonant with his dignity as a person.[2]

4. Man has the right and the duty to protect the integrity of his body together with all of its bodily functions.
5. Any procedure potentially harmful to the patient is morally justified only insofar as it is designed to produce a proportionate good.
6. Ordinarily the proportionate good that justifies a medical or surgical procedure should be the total good of the patient himself.
7. Adequate consultation is recommended, not only when there is doubt concerning the morality of some procedure, but also with regard to all procedures involving serious consequences, even though such procedures are listed here as permissible. The health facility has the right to insist on such consultations.
8. Everyone has the right and the duty to prepare for the solemn moment of death. Unless it is clear, therefore, that a dying patient is already well-prepared for death as regards both spiritual and temporal affairs, it is the physician's duty to inform him of his critical condition or to have some other responsible person impart this information.
9. The obligation of professional secrecy must be carefully fulfilled not only as regards the information on the patients' charts and records but also as regards confidential matters learned in the exercise of professional duties. Moreover, the charts and records must be duly safeguarded against inspection by those who have no right to see them.
10. The directly intended termination of any patient's life, even at his own request, is always morally wrong.
11. From the moment of conception, life must be guarded with the greatest care. Any deliberate medical procedure, the *purpose* of which is to deprive a fetus or an embryo of its life, is immoral.[3]
12. Abortion, that is, the directly intended termination of pregnancy before viability, is never permitted nor is the directly intended destruction of a viable fetus. Every procedure whose sole immediate effect is the termination of pregnancy before viability is an abortion, which in its moral

context, includes the interval between conception and implantation of the embryo.

13. Operations, treatments, and medications, which do not directly intend termination of pregnancy but which have as their purpose the cure of a proportionately serious pathological condition of the mother, are permitted when they cannot be safely postponed until the fetus is viable, even though they may or will result in the death of the fetus. If the fetus is not certainly dead, it should be baptized.
14. Regarding the treatment of hemorrhage during pregnancy and before the fetus is viable: Procedures that are designed to empty the uterus of a living fetus still effectively attached to the mother are not permitted; procedures designed to stop hemorrhage (as distinguished from those designed precisely to expel the living and attached fetus) are permitted insofar as necessary, even if fetal death is inevitably a side effect.
15. Caesarean section for the removal of a viable fetus is permitted, even with risk to the life of the mother, when necessary for successful delivery. It is likewise permitted, even with risk for the child, when necessary for the safety of the mother.
16. In extrauterine pregnancy the dangerously affected part of the mother (e.g., cervix, ovary, or Fallopian tube) may be removed, even though fetal death is foreseen, provided that (*a*) the affected part is presumed already to be so damaged and dangerously affected as to warrant its removal, and that (*b*) the operation is not just a separation of the embryo or fetus from its site within the part (which would be a direct abortion from a uterine appendage); and that (*c*) the operation cannot be postponed without notably increasing the danger to the mother.
17. Hysterectomy, in the presence of pregnancy and even before viability, is permitted when directed to the removal of a dangerous pathological condition of the uterus of such serious nature that the operation cannot be safely postponed until the fetus is viable.

B. PROCEDURES INVOLVING REPRODUCTIVE ORGANS AND FUNCTIONS

18. Sterilization, whether permanent or temporary, for men or for women, may not be used as a means of contraception.[4]
19. Similarly excluded is every action which, either in anticipation of the conjugal act, or in its accomplishment, or in the development of its natural consequences, proposes, whether as an end or as a means, to render procreation impossible.[5]
20. Procedures that induce sterility, whether permanent or temporary, are permitted when: (*a*) they are immediately directed to the cure, diminution, or prevention of a serious pathological condition and are not directly contraceptive (that is, contraception is not the purpose), and (*b*) a simpler treatment is not reasonably available. Hence, for example, oophorectomy or irradiation of the ovaries may be allowed in treating carcinoma of the breast and metastasis therefrom; and orchiectomy is permitted in the treatment of carcinoma of the prostate.[6]
21. Because the ultimate personal expression of conjugal love in the marital act is viewed as the only fitting context for the human sharing of the divine act of creation, donor insemination and insemination that is totally artificial are morally objectionable. However, help may be given to a normally performed conjugal act to attain its purpose. The use of the sex faculty outside the legitimate use by married partners is never permitted even for medical or other laudable purpose, e.g., masturbation as a means of obtaining seminal specimens.
22. Hysterectomy is permitted when it is sincerely judged to be a necessary means of removing some serious uterine pathological condition. In these cases, the pathological condition of each patient must be considered individually and care must be taken that a hysterectomy is not performed merely as a contraceptive measure, or as a routine procedure after any definite number of Caesarean sections.

23. For a proportionate reason, labor may be induced after the fetus is viable.
24. In all cases in which the presence of pregnancy would render some procedure illicit (e.g., curettage), the physician must make use of such pregnancy tests and consultation as may be needed in order to be reasonably certain that the patient is not pregnant. It is to be noted that curettage of the endometrium after rape to prevent implantation of a possible embryo is morally equivalent to abortion.
25. Radiation therapy of the mother's reproductive organs is permitted during pregnancy only when necessary to suppress a dangerous pathological condition.

C. OTHER PROCEDURES

26. Therapeutic procedures which are likely to be dangerous are morally justifiable for proportionate reasons.
27. Experimentation on patients without due consent is morally objectionable, and even the moral right of the patient to consent is limited by his duties of stewardship.
28. Euthanasia ("mercy killing") in all its forms is forbidden. The failure to supply the ordinary means of preserving life is equivalent to euthanasia. However, neither the physician nor the patient is obliged to the use of extraordinary means.[7]
29. It is not euthanasia to give a dying person sedatives and analgesics for the alleviation of pain, when such a measure is judged necessary, even though they may deprive the patient of the use of reason, or shorten his life.
30. The transplantation of organs from living donors is morally permissible when the anticipated benefit to the recipient is proportionate to the harm done to the donor, provided that the loss of such organ(s) does not deprive the donor of life itself nor of the functional integrity of his body.
31. Post-mortem examinations must not be begun until death is morally certain. Vital organs, that is, organs necessary to sustain life, may not be removed until death has taken place. The determination of the time of death must be made

in accordance with responsible and commonly accepted scientific criteria. In accordance with current medical practice, to prevent any conflict of interest, the dying patient's doctor or doctors should ordinarily be distinct from the transplant team.

32. Ghost surgery, which implies the calculated deception of the patient as to the identity of the operating surgeon, is morally objectionable.
33. Unnecessary procedures, whether diagnostic or therapeutic, are morally objectionable. A procedure is unnecessary when no proportionate reason justifies it. *A fortiori,* any procedure that is contra-indicated by sound medical standards is unnecessary.

SECTION II: THE RELIGIOUS CARE OF PATIENTS

34. The administration should be certain that patients in a health facility receive appropriate spiritual care.
35. Except in cases of emergency (i.e., danger of death), all requests for baptism made by adults or for infants should be referred to the chaplain of the health facility.
36. If a priest is not available, anyone having the use of reason and proper intention can baptize. The ordinary method of conferring emergency baptism is as follows: the person baptizing pours water on the head in such a way that it will flow on the skin, and while the water is being poured must pronounce these words audibly: *I baptize you in the name of the Father, and of the Son, and of the Holy Spirit.* The same person who pours the water must pronounce the words.
37. When emergency baptism is conferred, the chaplain should be notified.
38. It is the mind of the Church that the sick should have the widest possible liberty to receive the sacraments frequently. The generous cooperation of the entire staff and personnel is requested for this purpose.

39. While providing the sick abundant opportunity to receive Holy Communion, there should be no interference with the freedom of the faithful to communicate or not to communicate.
40. In wards and semiprivate rooms, every effort should be made to provide sufficient privacy for confession.
41. When possible, one who is seriously ill should be given the opportunity to receive the Sacraments of the Sick, while in full possession of his rational faculties. The chaplain must, therefore, be notified as soon as an illness is diagnosed as being so serious that some probability of death is recognized.
42. Personnel of a Catholic health facility should make every effort to satisfy the spiritual needs and desires of non-Catholics. Therefore, in hospitals and similar institutions conducted by Catholics, the authorities in charge should, with the consent of the patient, promptly advise ministers of other communions of the presence of their communicants and afford them every facility for visiting the sick and giving them spiritual and sacramental ministrations.[8]
43. If there is a reasonable cause present for not burying a fetus or member of the human body, these may be cremated in a manner consonant with the dignity of the deceased human body.[9]

September 1971. U.S.C.C.

NOTES

CHAPTER 1.
Surgery

1. June Goodfield, "Reflections on the Hippocratic Oaths," *The Hastings Center Studies*, vol. 1, no. 2 (1973): 81.
2. Richard A. McCormick, S.J., "Issue Areas for a Medical Ethics Program," in R. Veatch, ed., *The Teaching of Medical Ethics* (Hastings-on-Hudson: Hastings Center, 1973), pp. 106-107.
3. *Summa theologae* II-II, Ques. 65, Art. 1.
4. Cf., for instance, *Acta Apostolicae Sedis* (hereinafter referred to as AAS) 22 (1930) 565; 44 (1952) 782, 786-8; 45 (1953) 673-4, 747.
5. Gerald Kelly, S.J., "Artificial Means of Preserving Life," *Theological Studies* 11 (1950): 204-205.
6. Helmut Thielicke, "Ethische Fragen der modernen Medizin," *Archiv für klinische Chirurgie* 321 (1968): 13.
7. AAS 49 (1957) 1031-1032.
8. The pope said that one is held to use only ordinary means *normally*. No doubt he was thinking of two exceptions that moralists usually made to this rule: if a sinner had not yet reconciled himself with God, or if some individual's life were especially needed for the common good, he would have a duty to use extraordinary means because of the special circumstances.
9. Robert E. Rothenberg, M.D., *Understanding Surgery* (New York: Simon & Schuster, 1973), pp. 164 and 178.
10. Ibid., pp. 222 and 218.
11. John C. Ford, S.J., "The Refusal of Blood Transfusions by Jehovah's Witnesses," *Linacre Quarterly* 22 (1955): 3-10.
12. Paul Ramsey, *The Patient as Person* (New Haven: Yale University Press, 1970), p. 240.

13. *Chicago Sun-Times,* 26 March 1964, p. 42.
14. Ramsey, *Patient as Person,* p. 139.
15. Cf., e.g., Kelly, "Artificial Means of Preserving Life," pp. 212-213; and Edwin F. Healy, S.J., *Medical Ethics* (Chicago: Loyola University Press, 1956), p. 71.
16. Ramsey, *Patient as Person,* p. 139, no. 31.
17. Cf. above, pp. 4-7.
18. Quoted in the *Chicago Sun-Times,* 25 February 1974, p. 4.
19. *Chicago Sun-Times,* 25 February 1974, p. 16; and *Time,* 25 March 1974, p. 84.
20. *Time,* 25 March 1974, p. 84.
21. Charles McFadden, O.S.A., *Reference Manual for Medical Ethics* (Philadelphia: F. A. Davis Co., 1949), pp. 25-26.
22. Kelly, "Artificial Means of Preserving Life," pp. 211-212.
23. Ibid., p. 212, no. 277.
24. Ramsey, *Patient as Person,* pp. 131-132.
25. Healy, *Medical Ethics,* pp. 88-90.
26. Richard A. McCormick, S.J., "To Save or Let Die," *America,* 13 July 1974, pp. 6-10.
27. Healy, *Medical Ethics,* p. 89.
28. Ibid., pp. 69-70.
29. Ramsey, *Patient as Person,* p. 132.

CHAPTER 2.
Organ Transplantation

1. Paul Ramsey, *The Patient as Person* (New Haven: Yale University Press, 1970, p. 177.
2. Roberta G. Simmons and Julie Fulton, "Ethical Issues in Kidney Transplantation," in Claude A. Frazier, M.D., ed., *Is It Moral to Modify Man?* (Springfield, Ill.: Charles C. Thomas, 1973), p. 179.
3. Quoted in James B. Nelson, *Human Medicine* (Minneapolis: Augsburg Publishing House, 1973), p. 156.
4. David Daube, "Moral Problems in the Use of Borrowed Organs," *Annals of Internal Medicine* 60 (1964): 312.
5. AAS 22 (1930) 565.
6. AAS 44 (1952) 786.
7. Gerald Kelly, S.J., "Pius XII and the Principle of Totality," *Theological Studies* 16 (1955): 373-396.

8. Some efforts have been made to enlarge the meaning of the principle of totality to include organ transplantation. See, for instance, Martin Nolan, "The Principle of Totality in Moral Theology," in Charles Curran, ed., *Absolutes in Moral Theology?* (Washington: Corpus Books, 1968), pp. 232-248. Also, see the criticisms of this approach in Ramsey, *Patient as Person,* pp. 178-181.
9. Joseph Fletcher, "Our Shameful Waste of Human Tissue," in Donald R. Cutler, ed., *Updating Life and Death* (Boston: Beacon Press, 1969), p. 25.
10. Ramsey, *Patient as Person,* pp. 210-211.
11. AAS 45 (1957) 1027-1033.
12. Frank J. Ayd, M.D., "What is Death?" Unpublished address given at the Second National Council on Medical Ethics, sponsored by the Judicial Council of the American Medical Association, Oct. 5-6, 1968, Chicago, Illinois.
13. Paul Ramsey, "On Updating Death," in Cutler, *Updating Life and Death,* pp. 31-45. (Also, *Patient as Person,* pp. 59-112.).
14. Declaration of the World Medical Association meeting in Sydney, Australia, 7 August 1968.
15. Ad hoc committee of the Harvard Medical School, "A Definition of Irreversible Coma," *Journal of the American Medical Association* 205 (1968): 85-88.
16. Vincent J. Collins, M.D., "Limits of Medical Responsibility in the Prolongation of Life: A Guide to Decision—A Dying Score," *Journal of the American Medical Association* 206 (1968): 390.
17. Ramsey, *Patient as Person,* p. 66.
18. Simmons and Fulton, "Ethical Issues," p. 183.
19. Second National Council on Medical Ethics of the American Medical Association, Oct. 5-6, 1968, Chicago, Illinois.
20. 96, Cal. App. 2d 371, 211 P 2d 478.
21. Ad hoc committee of the Harvard Medical School, "A Definition of Irreversible Coma," p. 87.
22. Quoted in the *Chicago Sun-Times,* 22 May 1974, p. 58.
23. Simmons and Fulton, "Ethical Issues," p. 173.
24. David Sanders and Jesse Dukeminier, Jr., "Medical Advance and Legal Lag: Hemodialysis and Kidney Transplantation," *U.C.L.A. Law Review* 15 (1968): 378.

CHAPTER 3.
Human Experimentation

1. Cf., for example, M. H. Pappworth, M.D., *Human Guinea Pigs* (Boston: Beacon Press, 1967).
2. Henry K. Beecher, M.D., "Ethics and Clinical Research," *The New England Journal of Medicine* 274 (1966): 1355.
3. Henry K. Beecher, M.D., *Experimentation in Man* (Springfield, Ill.: Charles C. Thomas, n.d.), p. 43.
4. Paul Ramsey, *The Patient as Person* (New Haven: Yale University Press, 1970), pp. 6-7.
5. Hans Jonas, "Philosophical Reflections on Experimenting with Human Subjects," in Paul A. Freund, ed., *Experimentation with Human Subjects* (New York: George Braziller, 1970), p. 20.
6. Quoted in Henry K. Beecher, M.D., "Medical Research and the Individual," in Daniel H. Labby, ed., *Life or Death: Ethics and Options* (Seattle: University of Washington Press, 1968), pp. 128-129.
7. Ibid., p. 121.
8. Ibid., p. 131.

CHAPTER 4.
Contraception and Sterilization

1. Paul VI, *Humanae Vitae,* no. 11.
2. Ibid., no. 14.
3. Quoted in the *Chicago Sun-Times,* 18 April 1974, p. 17.
4. Address to the Planned Parenthood Affiliates, 15 May 1962.
5. Josef Fuchs, S.J., *De Castitate et Ordine Sexuali* (Rome: Gregorian University, 1960).
6. Paul VI, *Humanae Vitae,* no. 12.
7. Paul Ramsey, "A Christian Approach to the Question of Sexual Relations Outside of Marriage."
8. *Theological Studies* 29 (1968): 737.
9. Cf. Charles Curran, *New Perspectives in Moral Theology* (Notre Dame: Fides, 1974).

CHAPTER 5.
Transsexualism and Homosexuality

1. *Time,* 21 Jan. 1974, p. 63.
2. Charles J. McFadden, O.S.A., *Medical Ethics* (Philadelphia: F. A. Davis, 1967), p. 281.
3. Cf., for example, McFadden, *Medical Ethics,* pp. 279-283; Edwin F. Healy, S.J., *Medical Ethics* (Chicago: Loyola University Press, 1956), p. 135.
4. McFadden, *Medical Ethics,* p. 283.
5. Cf. above, chapter 4, p. 79.
6. Wardell B. Pomeroy, "Homosexuality," in Ralph W. Weltge, ed., *The Same Sex* (Philadelphia: Pilgrim Press, 1969), pp. 3-13.
7. John J. McNeil, S.J., "The Christian Male Homosexual," *Homiletic and Pastoral Review* 70 (1970): 667-677, 747-758, 828-836.
8. Charles E. Curran, "Dialogue with the Homophile Movement," *Catholic Moral Theology in Dialogue* (Notre Dame: Fides, 1972), pp. 184-219.

CHAPTER 6.
Genetic Manipulation

1. Long overlooked by scientists, DNA is now recognized as the basic ingredient of the gene. It is a double molecule—two long molecular strands twisted together. Each strand is made up of nucleotides, four different chemicals or bases —A (adenine), T (thymine), C (cytosine), and G (guanine)—which are strung together like beads on a chain. In human DNA there are about 1,000 million nucleotides, and they occur along the chain in a random selection of almost infinite variety. Hence, except for identical twins (or triplets, etc.), the DNA in each person is unique. The two strands are held together by hydrogen atoms which loosely join the nucleotides in each strand. Since A only combines with T, and C only combines with G, in cellular mitosis the DNA

splits down the middle and each base or nucleotide picks up its complementary base in the free-floating material in the new cell. The result is that in the new cell the DNA is exactly replicated. What is more, DNA directs the twenty different amino acids to produce the distinctive proteins which make up the various cells and organs of the human body. It imprints the appropriate message on a single-stranded chemical called RNA (ribonucleic acid), which carries the instructions to the protein-making substances. From DNA, the master blueprint, RNA delivers an exact copy for the formation of the cells of the various organs, e.g., heart, eyes, brain, lungs, etc. Since the DNA contains all the genetic information and is identical in every cell, it cannot be allowed to send out all its potential messages in every specialized cell. Certain enzymes are produced in the cells which turn on and off the appropriate switches. They produce certain repressors which cover over long segments of DNA in each cell and so prevent them from sending out those parts of their coded information that would be inappropriate in a certain specialized part of the organism.

There are only four letters in the genetic code (nucleotides A, T, G, and C). Combinations of three are necessary to make a "word," i.e., to effect the production of proteins. There are therefore sixty-four possible combinations, and researchers have isolated the combination necessary to call up and to shut off every amino acid in every living thing.

2. Cf. Isaac Asimov, *The Genetic Code* (New York: The New American Library, 1962).
3. See account of first documented case in Robert Francoeur, *Utopian Motherhood* (Garden City, N.Y.: Doubleday, 1970), pp. 1-3. Artificial insemination is achieved by injecting semen into the vagina with a syringe or by attaching a plastic cup containing semen to the cervix for about twenty-four hours.
4. Parthenogenesis has been accomplished by mechanical and electrical stimulation of an unfertilized egg cell, causing it to begin mitosis, but such cells have only a half complement of chromosomes and their development has not proceeded very far.

5. Gordon R. Taylor, *The Biological Time Bomb* (New York: The New American Library, 1969), pp. 214-215.
6. Quoted in Donald Fleming, "On Living in a Biological Revolution," *The Atlantic* 223 (1969): 67.
7. See Albert Rosenfeld, *The Second Genesis* (Englewood Cliffs, N.J.: Prentice-Hall, 1969), p. 117.
8. Francois Houtart, *The Eleventh Hour* (New York: Sheed and Ward, 1968), p. 46.
9. *Theological Studies* 30 (1969): 681.
10. James Gustafson, "Commentary on 'The Sanctity of Life,' " in Donald R. Cutler, ed., *Updating Life and Death* (Boston: Beacon Press, 1968), p. 232.
11. Helmut Thielicke, *The Ethics of Sex* (New York: Harper and Row, 1964), p. 199.
12. Paul Ramsey, *The Fabricated Man* (New Haven: Yale University Press, 1970).
13. Ibid. Ramsey notes some of the scientific and socio-psychological objection that could be raised: "(1) The genes of a supposedly superior male may contain injurious recessives which by artificial insemination would become widespread throughout the population instead of remaining in small proportion, as they now do; (2) the validity of this proposal is not demonstrated by the present-day children of geniuses; (3) it might turn out that parents who looked forward eagerly to having a Horowitz in the family would discover later that it was not so fine as they expected because he might have a temperament incompatible with that of a normal family, and it is bad enough if we take responsibility only for the environment of our children; if we take responsibility for their genetic make-up, too, the guilt may become unbearable; (4) we know nothing about the mutation rate that would continue in the frozen germ cells; (5) the I.Q.'s of criminals would be raised; (6) we could not have a 'healthy society' because not many men would be 'emotionally satisfied by children not their own' " (pp. 49-50).
14. Michael Hamilton, "New Life for Old: Genetic Decisions," *The Christian Century* 86 (1969): 743.
15. *Theological Studies* 30 (1969): 689.
16. Charles Curran, *Contemporary Problems in Moral Theology* (Notre Dame: Fides, 1970), p. 199.

17. *Collect. S.C. de Prop. Fide* II, n. 1964.
18. AAS 41 (1949) 559.
19. Ibid., 560.
20. AAS 43 (1951) 850.
21. *Theological Studies* 32 (1971): 97.
22. Roger Van Allen, "Artificial Insemination (AIH): A Contemporary Re-analysis," *Homiletic and Pastoral Review* 70 (1970): 363-372.
23. *Theological Studies* 30 (1970): 509.
24. Curran, *Contemporary Problems*, p. 213.
25. Professor Douglas Bevis of Leeds University recently claimed that three babies conceived in laboratory test tubes and then implanted in the mother's womb were born in Europe within the last eighteen months. See *Chicago Tribune*, 16 July 1974.
26. Quoted in Ramsey, *The Fabricated Man*, p. 73.
27. Karl Rahner, S.J., "Experiment: Man," *Theology Digest* 16 (1968): 57-69. (In "Zum Problem der genetischen Manipulation," *Schriften zur Theologie* 8, 286-321, Rahner shows himself to be considerably more conservative and cautious.)
28 H. Richard Niebuhr, *The Kingdom of God in America* (New York: Harper, 1937), p. 193.
29. P. B. Medawar, "Genetic Options," in Daniel H. Labby, ed., *Life or Death: Ethics and Options* (Seattle: University of Washington Press, 1968), p. 94.

CHAPTER 7.
Abortion

1. Exodus 21:22 requires that a man pay an appropriate fine if he accidentally causes a woman to have a miscarriage.
2. *Apologeticus* 9, 8.
3. *De Anima* 25, 4.
4. Cf. John F. Dedek, *Human Life* (New York: Sheed and Ward, 1972), pp. 38-40.
5. Ibid., pp. 41-42.
6. DS 2134-2135.
7. See ed. 7, vol. 2, tract. 2, cap. 3, n. 839-849.
8. In 1869 Pius IX dropped the distinction between an animated and nonanimated fetus in his reorganization of canon law.
9. *Summa theologae* II-II, 64, 7.

10. Antonius Ballerini, S.J., *Opus Theologicum Morale*, vol. 2, tract. 4, sect. 5, cap. 1, dub. 4; and *Compendium Theologiae Moralis*, Tom. I, tract. de Praecepto 5 Decalogi, cap. 2, art. 3.
11. Quoted in Lehmkuhl and Ballerini.
12. Quoted in Lehmkuhl and Ballerini.
13. The principle of double effect is generally enunciated something like this: it is morally permissible to place an action which has two foreseen effects, one good and one bad, if four conditions are all verified: (1) the action itself is good or indifferent; (2) the good effect is not produced by means of the bad effect; (3) only the good effect and not the bad effect is directly intended; (4) there is a proportionate reason for placing the action and permitting the bad effect.

    The *first condition* requires that the action itself be good or at least indifferent. The reason for this requirement is that if the action is morally wrong in itself, then it is already illicit independent of its consequences.

    The *second condition* requires that the good effect be not produced by means of the bad effect. The reason for this is that we may not do evil that good may come of it (Rom. 3:8). For to will evil as a means is to will it in itself if not for itself, and to deliberately will evil is morally wrong.

    To understand the implications of this second condition one should notice that the good and the evil effects can be related in three ways: (1) the action primarily produces the evil effect and the evil effect produces the good effect (example: a man in a burning building puts a loaded shotgun in his mouth and pulls the trigger so that he will avoid the pain of burning to death); (2) the action primarily produces the good effect and the good effect produces the bad effect (example: a surgeon saves the life of a despotic dictator and as a result his despotic rule continues); (3) the action produces both effects together and independently of each other (example: an aviator drops a bomb on a ship killing both combatants and innocent passengers). What is implied in this second condition is that numbers 2 and 3 can be licit but number 1 cannot.

    It is important to notice that the relation between the two effects that is relevant here is the relation of causality, not merely that of time. Temporal priority usually indicates a causal connection, but this is not necessarily the case. (Example: a surgeon removes a cancerous uterus containing a live, nonviable fetus. In order to remove the uterus he must first cut veins and arteries, thereby killing the fetus by severing its only lifelines. The death blow is first administered to the fetus chronologically before the womb is removed, and as a matter of fact the fetus is usually, though not always, dead before the uterus has been removed. Nonetheless, the same sealing of veins and arteries would be necessary even if there were no fetus present. Both effects issue from this act equi-immediately in the order of causality.) It is important to notice that the fact that the evil effect will certainly follow does not mean that it is the means to the good effect. (Example: the death of the fetus, although certain, is not the means to the mother's cure, but simply an inevitable effect of the hysterectomy.)

The *third condition* demands that only the good effect and not the evil effect be directly intended as the end of the action. For if evil is the end, the will embraces evil; that is to say, it deliberately chooses it.

The *fourth condition* is that there be a proportionate reason for placing the cause and permitting the evil effect. A proportionate reason is required to permit the foreseen evil because we are obliged not only not to intend or do evil, but also to avoid it insofar as it is morally possible to do so. A proportionate reason is sufficient to permit evil because if there is a proportionate reason, the avoidance of the evil is judged to be morally impossible and we are excused from the general obligation to avoid evil; that is to say, it is then reasonable to place the good act even though it has an unavoidable bad consequence.

14. DS 3258.
15. DS 3298.
16. DS 3336-3338.
17. Quoted in Lehmkuhl.
18. Paulist translation, n. 63-66.
19. Pius XII, AAS 43 (1951) 838-839.
20 *Gaudium et Spes*, n. 27.
21. Ibid., n. 51.
22. Paul VI, *Humanae Vitae*, 14.
23. Dietrich Bonhoeffer, *Ethics* (New York: Macmillan, 1965), p. 176.

24. Karl Barth, *Church Dogmatics*, vol. 3, part 4, p. 55.
25. Paul Ramsey, "The Morality of Abortion," in Daniel H. Labby, ed., *Life or Death: Ethics and Options* (Seattle: University of Washington Press, 1968), pp. 61-63.
26. Ibid., p. 63, no. 1.
27. Joseph Donceel, S.J., "Animation and Hominization," *Theological Studies* 31 (1970): 76-105.
28. Robert Springer, S.J., "Notes on Moral Theology," *Theological Studies* 31 (1970): 500-501.
29. Bernard Häring, *Medical Ethics* (Notre Dame: Fides, 1973), p. 101.
30. AAS (1951) 857.
31. AAS (1951) 838.
32. Bernard Häring, "A Theological Evaluation," in John T. Noonan, Jr., ed., *The Morality of Abortion* (Cambridge: Harvard University Press, 1970), pp. 136-137.
33. *Theological Studies* 31 (1970): 493.
34. Charles Curran, *Contemporary Problems in Moral Theology* (Notre Dame: Fides, 1970), pp. 144-145.
35. Charles Curran, *New Perspectives in Moral Theology* (Notre Dame: Fides, 1974), p. 191.
36. Richard McCormick, S.J., "Notes on Moral Theology," *Theological Studies* 35 (1974): 354.
37. Ibid.
38. Cf. ad hoc Committee on Pro Life Activities, National Conference of Catholic Bishops, "Pastoral Guidelines for the Catholic Hospital and Catholic Health Care Personnel," (Washington, D.C.: United States Catholic Conference, 1973).

CHAPTER 8.
Euthanasia

1. John Farrell, M.D., *The Journal of the South Carolina Medical Association* 54 (1957): 231-232.
2. Cf. K. Nolan, "The Problem of Care for the Dying," in Charles Curran, ed., *Absolutes in Moral Theology?* (Washington: Corpus Books, 1968), p. 125.
3. Margaret Mead, "The Cultural Shaping of the Ethical Situation," in Kenneth Vaux, ed., *Who Shall Live?* (Philadelphia: Fortress, 1970), p. 14.

4. Dietrich Bonhoeffer, *Ethics* (New York: Macmillan, 1965), pp. 160-166.
5. Karl Barth, *Church Dogmatics,* vol. 3, part 4, p. 55.
6. Paul Ramsey, "Reference Points in Deciding About Abortion," in John T. Noonan, Jr., ed., *The Morality of Abortion* (Cambridge: Harvard University Press, 1970), pp. 94-97.
7. Gerald Kelly, S.J., *Medico-Moral Problems* (St. Louis: The Catholic Hospital Association of the United States and Canada, 1958), p. 129.
8. Ibid.
9. Ibid.
10. Edwin F. Healy, S.J., *Medical Ethics* (Chicago: Loyola University Press, 1956), p. 68.
11. *Theological Studies* 11 (1950): 219-220.
12. Joseph Sullivan, *Catholic Teaching on the Morality of Euthanasia* (Washington: Catholic University of America Press, 1949), p. 72.
13. *Theological Studies* 11 (1950): 218.
14. Paul Ramsey, *The Patient as Person* (New Haven: Yale University Press, 1970), p. 130.
15. AAS 49 (1957) 1031-1032.
16. Ibid.
17. Bernard Bard and Joseph Fletcher, "The Right to Die," *The Atlantic,* January 1968, pp. 59-64
18. Pius XII, *Mystici Corporis,* n. 104.
19. Joseph Fletcher, *Morals and Medicine* (Boston: Beacon Press, 1954), pp. 172-210.
20. Ibid., pp. 187-188.
21. Quoted in Fletcher, *Morals and Medicine,* p. 202.
22. Bernard Häring, *Shalom: Peace. The Sacrament of Reconciliation* (New York: Farrar, Straus and Giroux, 1968), pp. 177-178.
23. Charles Curran, *Contemporary Problems in Moral Theology* (Notre Dame: Fides, 1970), p. 146.
24. Harmon Smith, *Ethics and the New Medicine* (Nashville: Abingdon, 1970), pp. 166-167.
25. A good summary of the current speculation and debate on this question can be found in Richard A. McCormick, S.J., "Notes on Moral Theology," *Theological Studies* 34 (1973): 53-102. See also Daniel C. Maguire, *Death By Choice* (Doubleday: Garden City, 1974); and Ramsey, *Patient as Person,* pp. 157-164.

CHAPTER 9.

Psychosurgery and Behavior Control

1. Elliot S. Valenstein, *Brain Control* (New York: John Wiley & Sons, 1974), p. 317.
2. Ibid., pp. 317-318.
3. Ibid., p. 99.
4. Steven Rose, *The Conscious Brain* (New York: Alfred A. Knopf, 1973), p. 296.
5. Vernon H. Mark, "Brain Surgery in Aggressive Epileptics," *The Hastings Center Report* 3, no. 1 (1973): p. 2.
6. Gerald Kelly, S.J., *Medico-Moral Problems* (St. Louis: The Catholic Hospital Association of the United States and Canada, 1958), p. 281.
7. *Ethical and Religious Directives for Catholic Hospitals* (St. Louis: The Catholic Hospital Association of the United States and Canada, 1949).
8. William Beecher Scoville, M.D., "Only as a Last Resort . . .," *The Hastings Center Report* 3, no. 1 (1973): p. 3.
9. Vernon H. Mark, M.D., "Brain Surgery in Aggressive Epileptics," *The Hastings Center Report* 3, no. 1 (1973): p. 2.
10. Ibid., p. 4.
11. Ibid., p. 4.
12. Ibid., pp. 2-3.
13. Valenstein, *Brain Control*, p. 339.
14. Scoville, "Only as a Last Resort . . .," p. 5.
15. London, 1949.

Notes to Appendix A

1. Washington, D.C.: United States Catholic Conference, 1971.
2. Of the two, the term "directives" seems preferable; but the term "code," which is used both officially and unofficially, is to some extent appropriate, since the bishops have presented ethical standards in codified form, the norms are given a legalist explanation in the preamble, and this "code" also has institutional implications which are singled out for special emphasis by the bishops. In this report both terms are used in reference to the same document.
3. This report does not offer bibliographical documentation beyond a few minimal references because of the nature and

purpose of the document and the inter-relation of the themes treated. This is not a scientific monograph intended for a single group of specialists or scholars, but the scholarly report of a study commission which has been drawn up for consideration by several publics. It draws on multiple expertise, extensive study, and broad consultation. Explanations of the development of many of the themes treated here have been amply offered elsewhere and in many cases are well known. Because the bibliographical and scholarly needs of the various professions will vary, this commission will welcome requests for background readings in any of the themes treated in this report.

4. For a detailed and informative analysis of the changing situation of Catholic sponsored health care facilities in a time of rapid social and cultural transformation, see *Study of the Future Role of Health Care Facilities under Catholic Auspices in the United States* (CHA Task Force, Phase II Report, Findings and Summary), (St. Louis: The Catholic Hospital Association, 1969).
5. *The Documents of Vatican II,* Walter M. Abbott and Joseph Gallagher, eds., (New York: Guild Press/American Press/Association Press, 1966) pp. 675-696.
6. Ibid., 341-366.
7. Ibid., 199-308.
8. Ottawa: The Catholic Hospital Association of Canada, 1970.
9. *Ethical and Religious Directives for Catholic Hospitals* (St. Louis: The Catholic Hospital Association, 1955) par. 3.
10. Cf. *Declaration on Religious Freedom,* par. 7.
11. Ibid., par. 3.
12. *Constitution on the Church,* par. 25.
13. Warren T. Reich, S.T.D., Chairman, is Senior Research Scholar, Kennedy Center for Bioethics, Georgetown University, Washington, D.C.: George D. Shoup, S.J., B.D., Ph.D., is an M.D. cand. at Yale University Medical School; Robert H. Springer, S.J., S.T.D., is Associate Professor of Christian Ethics, Woodstock College, New York; James A. O'Donohoe, J.C.D., is Professor of Moral Theology, St. John's Seminary, Brighton, Mass. and Visiting Lecturer at Harvard Divinity School; J. Bryan Hehir, Th.D. cand., Harvard Divinity School, is Lecturer in Theological Ethics, St. John's Seminary, Brighton, Mass; Margaret A. Farley, R.S.M., Ph.D., is Assis-

tant Professor of Ethics, Yale University Divinity School; Charles E. Curran is Professor of Moral Theology, Catholic University of America, Washington, D.C.; André E. Hellegers, M.D., is Professor of Obstetrics and Gynecology, Georgetown University Medical Center; George A. Kanoti, S.T.D., is Associate Professor of Christian Ethics, John Carroll University, Cleveland; Kieran Nolan, O.S.B., S.T.D., is Interdisciplinary Research Associate, The Institute of Religion, Texas Medical Center, Houston. Consultants to the Commission were Richard A. McCormick, S.J., S.T.D., Professor of Moral Theology, Bellarmine School of Theology, Chicago; and LeRoy Walters, Ph.D., Director, Kennedy Center for Bioethics, Georgetown University.

Notes to Appendix C

1. Vatican II: *Constitution on the Church*, no. 27.
2. *Pacem in Terris*, no. 11.
3. Vatican II: *The Church Today*, no. 51.
4. *Humanae Vitae*, no. 14.
5. *Humanae Vitae*, no. 14.
6. *Humanae Vitae*, no. 15.
7. Vatican II: *The Church Today*, no. 27.
8. Directory for the Application of the Decisions of the Second Ecumenical Council of the Vatican Concerning Ecumenical Matters, no. 63.
9. *Canon Law Digest*, vol. 6, p. 669.

INDEX

C

D

E

V

W

X

Z

Father John Dedek, Professor of Moral Theology at St. Mary of the Lake Seminary in Mundelein, Illinois, conducted the first ecumenical seminar in medical ethics for the Association of Chicago Theological Schools.

Born in Chicago, Father Dedek received his doctorate in sacred theology in 1958. He was associate editor at the *Chicago Studies* for thirteen years and the associate pastor of a suburban parish in Illinois for seven years. Fr. Dedek lectured at a medical convention in the Northwest United States and has conducted seminars for priests and chaplains in over twenty-five U.S. dioceses and in Asia. He has written numerous articles for various journals and is the author of many popular books such as *Contemporary Sexual Morality*, *Human Life: Some Moral Issues* and *Titius and Bertha Ride Again*.